DISCARDED

Women Over 50
Psychological Perspectives

Women Over 50
Psychological Perspectives

Edited by

Varda Muhlbauer
Netanya Academic College
Netanya, Israel

and

Joan C. Chrisler
Connecticut College
New London, Connecticut, USA

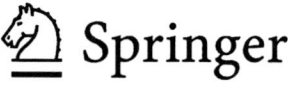

Varda Muhlbauer
Netanya Academic College
Kiryat Yitzhak Rabin
1 University Street
Netanya, 42365, Israel
Email: vardam@netvision.net.il

Joan C. Chrisler
Department of Psychology
Connecticut College
270 Mohegan Avenue
New London, CT 06320
USA
Email: jcchr@conncoll.edu

Library of Congress Control Number: 2006938388

ISBN-10: 0-387-46340-7
ISBN-13: 978-0-387-46340-7
eISBN: 978-0-387-46341-4

Printed on acid-free paper.

© 2007 Springer Science+Business Media, LLC

All rights reserved. This work may not be translated or copied in whole or in part without the written permission of the publisher (Springer Science+Business Media, LLC., 233 Spring Street, New York, NY 10013, USA), except for brief excerpts in connection with reviews or scholarly analysis. Use in connection with any form of information storage and retrieval, electronic adaptation, computer software, or by similar or dissimilar methodology now known or hereafter developed is forbidden.

The use in this publication of trade names, trademarks, service marks and similar terms, even if they are not identified as such, is not to be taken as an expression of opinion as to whether or not they are subject to proprietary rights.

9 8 7 6 5 4 3 2 1

springer.com

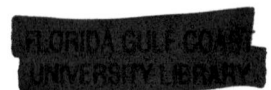

Foreword

It is truly remarkable that so little has happened in feminist studies in the last 20 years to rectify the dearth of psychological literature on older women. So it is with great pleasure that I note the publication of this book, which addresses so many of the needs that have gone begging for so long. But before I go forward to laud this volume, I'd like to go back in time to my own first reckonings that there was a great gap in the developmental story related to women's lives.

As I celebrated my 40th birthday and finished my graduate studies in the late 1970s, I became especially sensitive to the issue of women and aging. I was embarking on my dissertation research, which involved studying people between the ages of 65 and 100, most of whom were women, who were living either in their own homes, in retirement villages, or in nursing homes. As I did my literature review, I was struck by the paucity of research on women once they had reached a certain age. Like old soldiers, older women just seemed to fade away. From the time they had left puberty and found a life mate, the developmental psychology story had fewer and fewer episodes in each succeeding decade. What little was written tended to focus on loss—appearance, reproductive capacities, meaningful activity, sexual interest, mental stability, marital relationships, and, finally, cognitive capacities. Women were said to endure the pain of the "empty nest," menopause, loneliness, widowhood, and depression. It seemed that there was nothing nice to say; so why say much of anything at all?

In 1990 I wrote my article "Finished at 40" as a way of headlining the lack of presence of maturing women in the psychology literature. The title characterized the absence of both research and theory related to women's lives and also the perception that women's growth and development had already stopped by age 40. They were simply "finished," that is "used up," in the vernacular meaning of the word. Although I knew that there was some hyperbole in my framing of the title, I wanted the thesis to be provocative and to incite action. I hoped that feminist psychologists (and others) would pay more attention to older women's lives, and, most especially, I wanted more favorable, creative, and productive images cast for them.

As I myself was entering into this supposedly bleak and endless tunnel of loss, I recognized strong and contrary feelings of energy and potential within me. I wasn't going downhill; I was going up. Indeed I was about to enter a wonderful new phase of my professional life. And I was not alone. Around me were my friends and colleagues who were, for the most part, also vigorous, creative, and enthusiastic about their lives. Also reinforcing this alternative vision for what women might be were the data from my dissertation research. When asked what their most wonderful time of life was, the overwhelming choice for my women respondents was age 55. They loved that time, they said, because of their freedom from worry and the need to care for children and husbands; they described their lives at 55 as full of wealth, health, and activities galore. Some of them had interesting jobs; many had leadership roles in religious, civic, and social organizations. They traveled, learned new skills, and seemed to have a great deal of fun. Many relished the fact that worries about getting pregnant were behind them, and they spoke enthusiastically about their happy marriages, their grown-up children, and, most especially, their grandchildren. Most of the women in my study continued to have rewarding, active, and satisfying lives, although there were more challenges as they reached their 70s, 80s, and 90s. I recall, however, that two of the most interesting and intellectually lively participants were 90 and 100 years old, respectively.

Another research project involving women in their late 40s substantiated my view that life was getting better, not worse. As part of a study of the de-medicalization of menopause among the "patients-in-waiting," I asked women about their mood states at ages 20, 35, and at the present. For all of the participants, the least satisfying time of their lives was age 35 (Gergen, 1989). Apparently being a "soccer mom" was not the wonderful period of life that some might imagine. It helped to have a station wagon, but it didn't take away the longing to be free of some of the daily obligations that conspired against one's sense of having a personal identity or a personal life. Most were happy to have their children growing up, although they did anticipate the future with some trepidation; this was often brought about by their exposure to medical information about menopause and aging.

Today, I think if I could change the title of my article, it would be "Finished at 50," in that menopause is now the more common marker for the disappearance act. I might even be more optimistic and delete "finished" altogether. Since that article was published, the public, developmental psychologists, and gerontologists alike have concurred that 50 is the new 40; 60 is the new 50, etc. Middle age has been extended as well, and nobody wants to claim they are old anymore. There are many reasons for this recalibration, including better health care, "the pill," cosmetic surgery, women's liberation from certain social expectations (thanks to the feminist movement to a great extent), and a greater public acceptance of gender equality, especially in the workplace. There is an expansion of women's roles to include a professional life as well as a family one. The "social clock" of which Neugarten (1979) spoke has lost its Greenwich standard time. Parenting has become a multigenerational activity, as have attaining educational diplomas and changing career choices. Even sexual orientation is open for reconsideration in later years. One's social credit, at least for middle and upper middle class people, is, I think, enhanced by the denunciation of "traditional roles." Recently a friend of mine got remarried, took her husband on an adventure tour to Egypt to celebrate his 75th birthday, and became the head of her condominium board, all while pursuing her career as a painter; another has used her legal skills to adopt a child from Europe at age 53; a third, a new grandmother, has quit her job as a doctor to spend some time training horses and improving her dressage skills with her daughter. In all of these cases, middle age has only given these women the courage to engage in life to the fullest.

An exciting aspect of *Women Over 50: Psychological Perspectives* is that editors Varda Muhlbauer and Joan Chrisler, are advancing similar viewpoints, sharing with readers how blurred the age-group boundaries are and how women are defying limiting role expectations. Another important virtue of this volume is that, in itself, it creates a new climate for considering the meaning of aging. As people are exposed to this message, they become more open to re-evaluating their own lives and those of others with whom they live and work. Every promotion of this more positive vision of aging is critical in shifting a formerly devastating stereotype of the aging woman to one that is much more optimistic and powerful. In my own case, I am editing an electronic newsletter called the *Positive Aging Newsletter* (www.positiveaging.net) with Kenneth J. Gergen; in it we have set about reconstructing the stereotype of aging so that it is a time of generativity and strength. Instead of a downward spiral from a good life in youth and young adulthood, through middle age, to old age, and finally to death, we redefine aging as having an upward trajectory. To bolster our vision, we include material gathered from the social and biological sciences, as well as from news articles, Web sites, and books that find benefits and potentials in aging. Let others advertise the deficit discourses; that's not for us.

For me, "Finished at 40" was a clarion call for what I hoped would be a whole new world of research and theory making within the psychological community. At last, 16 years later, there seems to be a response. *Women Over 50: Psychological Perspectives* is elaborating the benefits, as well as the challenges, to women as they age. The authors advance the idea that this segment of the population should be taken seriously in terms of their political and social power. They are not simply patients waiting for the worst to befall them. Although it is extremely difficult to shake the prevailing problem-centered approach to aging, I commend the authors on their efforts, and wish them great success in this venture, now and in future editions. I also thank the editors for inviting me to write this foreword, which has encouraged me to reflect on this crucial period in my own development as a scholar and as a woman.

Mary Gergen

References

Gergen, M. (1989). Talking about menopause: A dialogic analysis. In L. E. Thomas (Ed.), *Research on adulthood and aging: The human sciences approach* (pp. 65–87). Albany, NY: State University of New York Press.

Gergen, M. (1990). Finished at 40: Women's development within the patriarchy. *Psychology of Women Quarterly, 14*, 471–493.

Neugarten, B. (1979). Time, age, and the life cycle. *American Journal of Psychiatry, 136*, 887–894.

Contents

Contributors xi

Introduction 1
Varda Muhlbauer and Joan C. Chrisler

1. Body Image Issues of Women Over 50 6
   Joan C. Chrisler

2. Women and Sex at Midlife: Desire, Dysfunction, and Diversity 26
   Maureen C. McHugh

3. Living Longer, Healthier Lives 53
   Susan D. Lonborg and Cheryl B. Travis

4. On the Move: Exercise, Leisure Activities, and Midlife Women 79
   Ruth L. Hall

5. The Well-being and Quality of Life of Women Over 50: A Gendered-Age Perspective 95
   Varda Muhlbauer

6. Enjoying the Returns: Women's Friendships After 50 112
   Suzanna M. Rose

7. Contemporary Midlife Grandparenthood 131
   Liat Kulik

8. Women Over 50: Caregiving Issues 147
   Rosalie J. Ackerman and Martha E. Banks

9. Work and Retirement: Challenges and Opportunities for
   Women Over 50 164
   Judith A. Sugar

10. Empowerment: A Prime Time for Women Over 50 182
    Florence L. Denmark and Maria D. Klara

Index 204

Contributors

Rosalie J. Ackerman is a clinical and research neuropsychologist and adjunct Professor of Clinical Psychology at Capella University. She has published many dozens of articles and book chapters, and she developed an award-winning Web site of resources for victims of domestic violence. She is best known for her work on intimate partner violence, rehabilitation of patients across the lifespan, and neuropsychological assessment, and she was instrumental in the development and revision of the Ackerman–Banks Neuropsychological Rehabilitation Battery and the Post-Assault Traumatic Brain Injury Interview & Checklist.

Martha E. Banks is a research neuropsychologist, retired clinical psychologist, and former Professor of Black Studies at the College of Wooster. She has authored dozens of articles and book chapters on violence against women, women with disabilities, ethnic minority women's concerns, and neuropsychological assessment and treatment, and she was instrumental in the development and revision of the Ackerman-Banks Neuropsychological Rehabilitation Battery and the Post-Assault Traumatic Brain Injury Interview & Checklist. She is co-editor of the book *Women with Visible and Invisible Disabilities: Multiple Intersections, Multiple Issues, Multiple Therapies*.

Joan C. Chrisler is Professor of Psychology at Connecticut College, where she teaches courses on the psychology of women and health psychology. She has published dozens of journal articles and book chapters on women's health and embodiment, and she is particularly known for her work on menstruation and menopause, autoimmune disorders, body image, weight, and eating disorders. She has served as editor of *Sex Roles: A Journal of Research*, and among her previous books are *From Menarche to Menopause: The Female Body in Feminist Therapy*, *Lectures on the Psychology of Women*, and *Arming Athena: Career Strategies for Women in Academe*.

Florence L. Denmark is the Robert Scott Pace Distinguished Research Professor at Pace University. She has published dozens of articles, books, and book chapters on the psychology of women and social psychology, and she is best known for her work on women's leadership and leadership styles, the interaction of status and gender, aging in cross-cultural perspective, and the contributions of women to psychology. She has held leadership roles in many professional organizations, including a term as president of the American Psychological Association, and is currently the main NGO representative to the United Nations for both the APA and the International Council of Psychologists. Her most recent books are *Engendering Psychology: Women and Gender Revisited*, *Violence in the Schools: Cross-national and Cross-cultural Perspectives*, and *International Perspectives on Violence*.

Mary Gergen is Professor Emerita of Psychology and Women's Studies at Pennsylvania State University—Delaware County. She has published extensively on the psychology of women, narrative psychology, aging, and research methodologies. Her most recent books are *Feminist Reconstruction in Psychology: Narrative, Gender, and Performance* and *Social Construction: Entering the Dialogue*. She and her husband Kenneth J. Gergen currently edit the *Positive Aging Newsletter*.

Ruth Hall is Professor of Psychology at The College of New Jersey. She is a sport psychologist and a licensed clinical psychologist. She is known for her research and writing on sport and exercise, African American women, and sexual orientation. She is co-editor of the book *Exercise and Sport in Feminist Therapy: Constructing Modalities and Assessing Outcomes*.

Maria D. Klara is a doctoral candidate in clinical child psychology at Pace University, where she serves as Florence Denmark's graduate assistant. Her clinical experience is working with children and their families, and her research interests include empowerment, resilience, and the role of grandparents in family dynamics.

Liat Kulik is Associate Professor of Social Work at Bar Ilan University. She has published extensively on gendered aspects of every day life, and she is best known for her work on power relations within the family, gender roles at work and at home, work–family conflict, and the intergenerational transmission of attitudes.

Susan Lonborg is Professor of Psychology at Central Washington University, where she teaches courses in health psychology, counseling, ethics, and the psychology of gender. She has published extensively in her areas of interest: applied health psychology, counseling processes and outcomes, and women's career development.

Maureen C. McHugh is Professor of Psychology at Indiana University of Pennsylvania, where she teaches courses on the psychology of women and social psychology. She has published dozens of articles and book chapters on gender issues, and she is best known for her work on gender differences, feminist methodologies and pedagogies, violence against women, and women's sexuality. She recently co-edited special issues on gender and violence for *Sex Roles* and *Psychology of Women Quarterly*.

Varda Muhlbauer is a senior Lecturer in the Department of Management and Business Administration at the Netanya Academic College, Israel. She has worked extensively over many years in teaching, researching, and consulting regarding women's issues from a feminist perspective. She was among the initiators of a pioneering center in Israel that conducted programs designed to advance women in the workplace and to aid women in distress. The center was based on principles of feminist social psychology and utilized cognitive–behavioral interventions.

Suzanna Rose is Professor of Psychology and Director of Women's Studies at Florida International University, where she teaches courses on gender and social psychology. She has published dozens of articles and book chapters, and she is best known for her work on friendship, love scripts, gay and lesbian issues, and the ways that gender, sexual orientation, and race affect interpersonal relationships. The advice contained in her book *Career Guide for Women Scholars* has contributed to the success of many women faculty.

Judith A. Sugar is Associate Professor of Public Health at the University of Nevada—Reno, where she teaches courses on aging. As a life span developmental psychologist, she has published dozens of articles and book chapters on aging, cognition, and health, and she is best known for her work on quality of life in frail elders, aging and memory, faculty retirement, and gerontology education in universities and colleges. She has held many leadership roles in academia and professional organizations.

Cheryl Brown Travis is Professor of Psychology and Chair of the Women's Studies Program at the University of Tennessee—Knoxville, where she teaches courses on the psychology of gender and social psychology. She has published extensively on women's health issues, particularly medical practice patterns, equity, and quality of health care delivery. She authored a pioneering two-volume text on *Women and Health Psychology*; her most recent books are *Evolution, Gender, and Rape* and *Sexuality, Society, and Feminism*.

Introduction

Varda Muhlbauer and Joan C. Chrisler

The shift in the cultural representations and real life experiences of women at midlife is much more than a passing trend. Rather, it is the product of a substantial transformation in the sociocultural construction of collective gendered-age identity, which has given rise to a blurring and diversification of both age and gender roles. By moving away from the traditional sociocultural construct of middle-age, the newly evolving gendered-age representations of women over 50 have generated positive meanings and more liberal behavior codes. This is a welcome move toward a better-balanced representation of this age group of women.

As committed feminist researchers, we hold to the long-established claim that the existing political constellation (i.e., male supremacy), which is clearly indicative of an uneven balance of power, is at the core of the sociocultural representations of both gender and age. Indeed the connection cannot be overstated. Our thesis endorses Sampson's (1993) assertions that representations, as evidenced in the current discourse on power, constitute the foundations of what people have come to accept as reality. Thus, the reconstruction of gendered-age representations of women over 50, which defines a better and more equitable division of power and greater personal and collective freedom, ultimately may lead to a fundamentally changed reality.

The present cohort of women over 50 has benefited from the accomplishments achieved in the wake of the massive societal changes of the last four decades, including the feminist movement, the gay rights movement, and the sexual revolution of the 1960s and 1970s and the more recent fight against ageism (including the baby boomers' refusal to see themselves as aging). The feminist movement made major strides in the reconstruction of gender roles on a more egalitarian basis. This influential development facilitated the empowerment of women mainly through educational and professional gains (Barnett & Hyde, 2001). Currently, as part of the antiageist revolution, the empowered cohort of women in midlife is rewriting its own collective identity (Ashmore et al., 2004) and thus expanding its boundaries and experiences through discursive processes.

The current shift in the representations and lifestyles of middle-aged women is marked, and already has spawned what might be called "a new middle-aged collective identity." A quick Internet search revealed the ways in which women in midlife (a term with flexible boundaries) have differentiated themselves from "old women." Key words such as "elderly women" bring up different Web sites (often medically oriented) than do key words such as "middle-aged women" or "women over 50." It was a pleasant surprise to discover how many sites intended for women over 50 are concerned with romance, sex, friendship, and general joie de vivre. Some of the nonacademic sites relate to an active sexuality, which is almost de rigueur for this age group of women. The Internet thus provides a fine illustration of what Mitchell and Helson (1990) referred to as the prime of life.

Transformative sociocultural discourse also has been successful in shifting the focus away from menopause to other age-related issues. Moreover, menopause itself has been given alternative interpretations that tend to reflect more closely the authentic attitudes of women in this age group. Many women enjoy the new freedom and possibilities that are open to them with the termination of the reproductive phase of their lives. The fact that this is in sharp contrast to traditional perceptions of menopausal women is another product of the overall transformation of women's place in society.

Therefore, it comes as no surprise that women currently in midlife (however they define it) differ considerably from midlife women of previous generations. Personal recollections of our own mothers and other women in their generation readily confirm this change. When middle-aged women today look at photographs of their mothers, their response often is: "I can't be the same age now that she was in that picture ... she looks so much older." Of course, women of today are in better physical health and wear more youthful fashions than women of yesteryear, but the difference between us and our mothers is much more than meets the eye. We have experienced a psychological makeover facilitated by the sociocultural changes in gender equity.

It goes without saying that there is great variability within the generation that has been privileged to undergo the cultural transformation that has bettered the quality of our lives. Many women cannot claim achievements in power domains, either institutional or personal, and, consequently, in well-being. However, on the whole, aspects of the transformation seem to be inclusive enough to trigger the need to take the pulse of this generation and raise questions related to all pertinent spheres of women's lives. We must remain mindful of the fact that women in midlife—both collectively and individually—are being thrust into novel gendered-age roles for which they have little training and about which they have scant information. Therefore, we have invited feminist scholars to share their knowledge about midlife women and to help us to think through the sum of what we know, and what we need to learn, about the group at the center of this remarkable transformation.

The word "aging" typically brings to mind changes in the body—both superficial (e.g., gray hair, wrinkles) and organic (e.g., chronic illness, infirmity). Thus, we begin with several chapters that concern aspects of midlife women's embodiment. Joan Chrisler examines the available research on body image issues of women over 50. She finds that the research that exists is generally not specific to this age group and that how well or poorly women seem to adjust to age-related changes in their bodies may depend on how the data are acquired. There is a lot yet to be done to understand how satisfied midlife women are with their bodies and how to assist those who are dissatisfied to learn to care for and about their bodies more positively.

Maureen McHugh exposes myths and stereotypes about sex and romance at midlife. She shows readers how to consider women's sexuality in context and explains why it should not be measured by androcentric standards. Sexual urges and the need to give and receive affection do not disappear with age, and the evidence shows that all most women need to enjoy active sex lives is a willing and caring partner and their own ability to define for themselves what form lovemaking will take.

Midlife is a time when many chronic illnesses are first diagnosed, and some of those illnesses are more likely to be experienced by women than by men. Susan Lonborg and Cheryl Travis review some of the recent research on women's health at midlife and put that work in the context of medicine's historic neglect of women's health conditions. They offer a number of suggestions about the use of self-care to prevent the development (or worsening) of chronic illnesses.

Self-care includes fun as well as work. Ruth Hall encourages us all to remember that in her chapter on exercise and leisure activities. Exercise is an important form of physical illness prevention, and it also helps to keep us mentally alert and psychologically healthy. When today's midlife women were children it was considered unusual for girls and women to take up sports, and therefore we may have to struggle at first before we get to the point where we enjoy our daily exercise routines. If that sounds familiar, let Coach Hall give you a pep talk!

Exercise, sexual activity, and physical health all contribute to women's well-being and quality of life. Varda Muhlbauer shows us how expanded gender roles, empowerment, self-confidence, positive media images and messages, and the enhanced freedom of self-definition that more liberal lifestyles provide can impact the quality of life of middle-aged women. Women over 50 today have a greater opportunity than previous generations could imagine to determine the course of their lives and pursue their own aims. And we are seizing those opportunities!

Women's lives at any age include varied roles and relational contexts. Suzanna Rose examines the role of friendships in middle-aged women's lives. The end of childrearing often means more time to spend with friends, and, as we age, our friends often become more dear to us. Yet, until recently, women's friendships were a neglected topic of research, and, even now, we know less about friendship at midlife than we do about the role of friends in other age groups. Perhaps the existence of the Red Hat Society will spark an interest in this topic. Wouldn't that be an interesting group to study?

Grandmotherhood is a role many women eagerly await, and it is often experienced for the first time in midlife. Liat Kulik reviews the research on grandparenthood, often referred to as a "roleless role" because its rights and obligations are more open to interpretation than is true of many other roles. Some grandmothers rarely see their grandchildren and communicate with them infrequently via telephone or e-mail. Others live nearby and are an important part of their grandchildren's lives, especially at holidays or when last-minute babysitters are needed. Still others end up raising their grandchildren in their own homes. Little is known about how contemporary grandmothers might differ from grandmothers of previous generations in the way they create this role for themselves.

Midlife is often referred to as "the sandwich generation" because middle-aged women often have caregiving responsibilities for children still at home (or for grandchildren whose parents need help raising them) and for their own parents, who maybe ill or disabled. Rosalie Ackerman and Martha Banks provide poignant examples of busy midlife women whose lives were disrupted by the call to care for a friend or family member who needed their assistance. The acts of giving and receiving care are both beneficial and stressful. This chapter will help us to think through ways to prepare for the caregiving that most of us will have to give and receive as we age.

Midlife is usually the peak earning point of people's careers and the time when they accomplish the most. It is also the time when people begin to plan seriously for retirement. Judith Sugar explains why so little is known about women's retirement planning and adjustment—after all, we can never really "retire" from our traditional work as homemakers. She critiques the androcentric perspective of most of the available research and exposes the sexism in retirement policies. This chapter is a must read for any woman who hopes to retire, and it provides a blueprint for activism to promote greater equity for all working women.

The life experience and self-confidence that women have earned by the time they reach midlife are often experienced as empowering, and this empowerment can be used effectively to make positive changes in one's own life, in the lives of others around us, and in the larger society. Florence Denmark and Maria Klara review the feminist research on empowerment, explain how women can increase their empowerment by working collectively, and suggest ways that midlife women can use their empowerment for the public good. They provide inspiring examples of what some empowered women over 50 have accomplished.

We are delighted that Mary Gergen accepted our invitation to provide a preface, in which she reminisces about her own midlife empowerment and how it led to her work on positive aging. Her article "Finished at 40" (which she says she would call "Finished at 50" if she were writing it today!) is a feminist classic, and this book would probably not exist if she had not led the way. We thank all of the authors for their thought-provoking contributions to this volume; we have all learned a lot from each other's work. We hope that our readers will be inspired to expand the literature by filling in the blanks we have identified and discovering the answers to the questions we have raised. We look forward to reading the work to come and to finding out how future generations of women over 50 will live out their lives.

References

Ashmore, R.D., Deaux, K., and McLaughlin-Volpe, T. (2004). An organizing framework for collective identity: Articulation and significance of multidimensionality. *American Psychologist, 130*, 80–114.

Barnett, R.C., and Hyde, J.S. (2001). Women, men, work, and family. *American Psychologist, 56,* 781–796.

Gergen, M. (1990). Finished at 40: Women's development within the patriarchy. *Psychology of Women Quarterly, 14,* 471–493.

Mitchell, V., and Helson, R. (1990). Women's prime of life: Is it the 50s? *Psychology of Women Quarterly, 14,* 451–470.

Sampson, E.E. (1993). Identity politics: Challenges to psychology's understanding. *American Psychologist, 48,* 1219–1230.

1
Body Image Issues of Women Over 50

Joan C. Chrisler

> The CIA should hire as spies
> only women over fifty, because
> we are the truly invisible.
> (Piercy, 2006, p. 1)

In her poem *I Met a Woman Who Wasn't There*, Marge Piercy (2006) described a common sensation experienced by midlife women: the transition from visibility to invisibility. In cultures in which notions of beauty and femininity are closely tied to youth, there comes a point when women, no matter how healthy, well groomed, and nicely attired they are, can pass by without attracting the attention of men or younger women. The point at which this happens no doubt differs for different women, but anecdotal evidence suggests that it is around age 50 when women, particularly women who had previously been praised as beautiful, suddenly realize that no one is looking at them anymore. This realization is a shock, but then what happens? Some women seem to react with relief—there is no longer any need to dress up and make up in order to impress; they can relax and simply be themselves. Other women panic—those who can afford it seek out cosmetic surgeons, personal trainers, and others who earn a living that derives in large part from the fear of aging. Is there any way to predict which women will react which way? How do women feel about the changes that accompany aging? How well or poorly do they adjust to those changes? These are some of the topics this chapter will address.

Youth-oriented Cultures

It can be a challenge to feel comfortable about aging in cultures where older women are rarely seen, and those who are seen are celebrated primarily for their "youthful" good looks (Chrisler & Ghiz, 1993). Although we are told that we are only as old as we feel, the dearth of images of women over 50 in the media drive home the message that women should either grow old "gracefully" by hiding the signs of aging (Chrisler & Ghiz, 1993) or stay out of sight. Wolf (1991) interviewed editors of North American women's magazines who admitted that signs of aging are routinely "airbrushed" from photographs through computer imaging, so that 60-year-old women are made to look 45. *Lear's*, a U.S. magazine aimed at midlife women (it's slogan was "the magazine for the woman who wasn't born yesterday"; it ceased publication after only a few years), rarely published photographs of gray-haired women (Gerike, 1990), and a content analysis (Nett, 1991) of *Chatelaine*, a Canadian magazine for midlife women, showed that midlife women were absent from the covers and the fashion and beauty sections and underrepresented in the advertisements. The editorial decisions made by the magazines' staff suggest that even midlife women do not want to see images of midlife women. Perhaps the editors are correct, but, if so, it is because the media shape women's preferences. Midlife women told McFarland (1999) that they are well aware that the media create the beauty standards women espouse; even though midlife women have the wisdom to realize that the images represent fantasy rather than reality, many of them still wish that they could match those standards.

Most women in Hollywood films are in their 20s and 30s (Lauzen & Dozier, 2005). It is not uncommon to see older men paired romantically on screen with women several decades younger than they are; for example, Clint Eastwood, Sean Connery, and Jack Nicholson have continued to play romantic lead roles well into their 70s. But as women approach midlife they begin to disappear from the Hollywood scene. Some who have had cosmetic surgery can hang on to their careers into their 40s, but eventually they find that there are few roles for them unless they start production companies and develop film projects for themselves. In the 2003 film *Something's Gotta Give* Diane Keaton played a woman in her 50s who stole her daughter's lover played by Jack Nicholson. It was both a shock and a delight to see Keaton on the screen—beautiful, yet clearly showing signs of age that had not been surgically altered. In a content analysis of the top 100 grossing Hollywood films of 2002, Lauzen and Dozier (2005) found that midlife and older women were seen on screen significantly less often than their male peers. As female characters aged, they were less likely to have goals or a purpose to their lives; as male characters aged, they were more likely to have power.

The same invisibility of midlife and older women is found on U.S. broadcast television. Over the years a number of content analyses (Gerbner et al., 1980; Glascock, 2001; Vernon et al., 1991) of prime time television programming have shown that the majority of female characters are 35 years old or younger, whereas male characters are more evenly distributed across the age range—at least up to the mid-50s. Davis (1990) found little gender difference in the number of female (12.1%) and male (14.8%) characters over age 50, but Vernon et al. (1991) pointed out that older men tend to be portrayed more positively than older women. The invisibility of older women is as common in news and public affairs programming as it is in entertainment programming. Former Secretary of State Madeline Albright is the only older woman I regularly see on these programs, and it is not unusual to find her on a panel with a number of men her age and older, usually being interviewed by male journalists over age 50. Barbara Walters has managed to continue her career well beyond the age when most women on television fade away, but she has had cosmetic surgeries over the years so that she does not look her age. Mike Wallace, Jim Lehrer, and other older men are able to continue their news careers as long as they like without altering their signs of aging, which are interpreted by viewers as indications of their wisdom and experience.

Women over 50 also are neglected in both popular and scholarly literature. Most books about midlife women are focused on menopause. A 1990 special issue of *Psychology of Women Quarterly (PWQ)* titled "Women at Midlife and Beyond" (edited by Violet Franks and Iris Fodor) was intended to encourage research on the many aspects of midlife and older women's lives. It is certainly true that more research is available now than when the issue was published, but much of what is available concerns women over 65. At the end of her 5 years as editor of *PWQ*, Jackie White (2005) looked back over the articles she had published and found that only 20% of those articles contained any data from women over 50. She concluded that women over 30 are an under-researched population. As I prepared to write this chapter I read a number of articles in which the body image of college students was compared to that of a convenience sample of older women. "Older women" was often broadly defined, for example, as women ages 30 to 84. It seems obvious that concerns of women in their 30s will differ (at least to some extent) from those of women in their 40s, 50s, 60s, 70s, and 80s, but how are we to tell what those differences are if researchers see any woman who is over 30 as "old"?

So what are women over 50 to think, and how are they to feel, about themselves if they cannot see other women their age in magazines and newspapers, in films and on television, or find their lives reflected in the contents of bookstore shelves or the pages of scholarly journals? The focus on menopause as the paramount issue of women in their 50s drives home the message that what is important about midlife is the end of youth and fertility. Once women have passed reproductive age, the culture seems to say, they are no longer interesting. No one cares about them. No one wants to see them or hear what they have to say. As Piercy (2006, p. 2) put it, "but to your prophecies only your cats will listen."

What Is Body Image?

Body image can be defined as individuals' appraisals of and feelings about their bodies and bodily functions (Cornwell & Schmitt, 1990). Body image is a cognition, an internal and subjective representation or map of physical appearance, sensation, motion, and other bodily experiences (Pruzinsky & Cash, 1990). It encompasses such aspects as weight consciousness; satisfaction or dissatisfaction with various parts of the body; proprioception, interoceptive awareness, balance, and other bodily sensations; understanding of one's skills and physical abilities; and adjustment to changes in the body that result from injury, aging, or illness. Body image is an important part of people's self-concept and, as such, provides a basis for our identity (Chrisler & Ghiz, 1993). It acts as a standard that influences not only the way we think about ourselves, but also our ability to perform various activities and the goals we set for the future (O'Brien, 1980). Although body image does not alter from day to day, it should not be considered fixed or static

(Pruzinsky & Cash, 1990). It develops throughout life as a result of maturation, sensory and behavioral experience, physical appearance, somatic changes, societal and cultural norms, and the reactions of other people (O'Brien, 1980).

Until recently psychological researchers have all but ignored body image issues of midlife and older women; most of their attention has been focused on adolescents and young adults, perhaps because of the connection between a poor body image and the development of eating disorders, or perhaps because researchers think that attractive and active bodies are more important to younger than to older people. The medical researchers who have investigated the topic have been primarily concerned with the impact of surgery or chronic illness on body image. Midlife is a time when people begin to be diagnosed in large numbers with chronic illnesses, so that is certainly an important topic to investigate, but it does not represent the only concern midlife women might have. Because of Western societies' creation of a strong beauty culture and insistence that women pursue an illusive beauty ideal (Freedman, 1986; Saltzberg & Chrisler, 1995; Wolf, 1991), because of the tendency in many societies to see youth and beauty as synonymous (Alderson, 1991), and because of the tendency to define woman as her body (Greenspan, 1983) or woman as her face (Sontag, 1979), one can expect to find women reporting body image concerns as they adjust to bodily changes that are concomitant with aging.

Weight Consciousness

The body's basal metabolic rate slows down with age, and is accompanied by a decrease in lean body tissue and an increase in fat (Rodin et al., 1984). A study (Young et al., 1963) of a large sample of midlife and older women showed an increase in body fat composition after age 50. The mean percentage of body fat in women in their 40s was 23%; it was 46% in women in their 50s, and 55% in women in their 60s. Women tend to gain weight at each of the major reproductive milestones (menarche, pregnancy, and menopause; Rodin et al., 1984), and the average age of menopause in North America is 51 years. Furthermore, weight may become redistributed during perimenopause, which results in larger breasts and waist and increased fat on the upper back (Voda et al., 1991). To put it simply, women should expect to gain weight and change shape as they get older, media ideals notwithstanding.

A number of researchers have reported weight-related concerns among midlife women. Wilcox (1996) surveyed women and men ages 20 to 80 about physical health status and attitudes toward their bodies. Older women with greater body mass index (BMI) reported more negative attitudes than did younger women or age peers with lower BMI. Donaldson (1994) surveyed 180 women ages 40 to 59, and found that weight status was the largest predictor of body image at midlife. Disparaging oneself and "feeling fat" were particularly related to the salience of body weight and shape, especially weight gain in the lower body. Lesbians were less concerned than straight women were about lower body fatness. McFarland (1999) conducted in-depth interviews with 10 midlife women about their body image at various points in their lives. The women frequently brought up weight gain and loss, which they seemed to see as evidence of their competence and their success or failure. Weight-related comments were made about both appearance and health concerns.

Markey et al. (2004) surveyed 172 midlife married couples in the northeastern United States for a study of family health. They reported that the wives were much more dissatisfied with their own bodies than the husbands were with their wives' bodies. The wives estimated that their husbands were much less satisfied than they actually were with their wives' appearance, and the wives selected a smaller body from the Figure Rating Scale (FRS) than their husbands did as the ideal for women their age. Wives' BMI was not strongly related to the husbands' satisfaction with their wives' bodies. This study is interesting in that it supports the results of previous studies (Fallon & Rozin, 1985; Miller, 2001; Rozin & Fallon, 1988) that have shown a discrepancy between what body size and shape men think is most attractive and what size and shape women think that men think is most attractive. Men generally choose a larger body size for women than women chose for themselves. If women allowed themselves to believe their partners when they say "You look fine to me," then women might feel more comfortable with body changes that occur at midlife.

Although eating disorders are usually associated with adolescent and young adult women, evidence of disordered eating has also been documented in midlife women. As the studies reviewed are all cross-sectional, it is impossible to tell whether the women in question had had eating disorders earlier in life or whether their disordered attitudes and behaviors emerged in midlife in reaction to age-related weight gain. Lewis and Cachelin (2001) reported that midlife women (ages 50 to 65) had higher scores on the Eating Disorders Inventory than did older women (ages 66 and older). They found positive correlations between fears of aging and attitudes and behaviors associated with disordered eating. Gupta and Schork (1993) also reported a direct connection between aging-related concerns and drive for thinness in a sample of 200 women (ages 30s to 50s) who were surveyed at a shopping mall.

However, not all midlife women hold themselves to unrealistic weight standards. Deeks and McCabe (2001) surveyed 304 women (ages 35 to 65) drawn from the community in and around Melbourne, Australia. The found that the premenopausal women selected smaller figures from the FRS than peri- and postmenopausal women did in response to a question about how society expected them to look. In a comparison of college students to a community sample of adults over age 39 from the southeastern United States, Lamb et al. (1993) found that women in both age groups would like to be thinner, but the young women chose a much thinner figure from the FRS as their ideal. These studies suggest that midlife women do not think that they are expected to measure up to the ideal weight standards to which younger women aspire. Furthermore, in a survey of 180 women (ages 18 to 60) Tiggemann and Stevens (1999) found that stronger feminist attitudes were correlated with lower weight concern, and Stevens et al. (1994) reported that the older Black women they surveyed were less likely than the older White women to consider themselves overweight. The White women also chose a smaller ideal body size on the FRS than the Black women did.

Body Esteem and Self-esteem

Body image is related to self-esteem in all age groups (Davidson & McCabe, 2005). Tiggemann and Stevens (1999) found that weight-related concerns predicted low self-esteem in women ages 30 to 49, but not in women over 50. Rackley et al. (1988) reported that high self-esteem and positive body image were correlated in a sample of midlife women. Other aspects that correlated with body image in their sample were feelings of self-worth, internal locus of control, and ratings of physical attractiveness. Stokes and Frederick-Recascino (2003) surveyed 144 U.S. women ages 18 to 87, and found no age-related differences in body esteem. They did, however, find that happiness predicted positive body esteem, which they measured as sexual attractiveness, weight concern, and physical condition. Related results were found by Fooken (1994) in her study of 60 German women ages 57 to 86. Those with a more positive body image had greater psychological well-being and were more likely than those with body image concerns to be sexually active. It is interesting to note that one of Fooken's body image measures was the question: "How do you feel about being naked and nakedness?"

A large literature (e.g., Chrisler & Lamont, 2002; Hays, 1999; Pettus, 2001) demonstrates the positive relations between physical activity and self-esteem and body image. However, women with poor body esteem often avoid activities (e.g., exercise) and situations that might improve their well-being (McLaren & Kuh, 2004). For example, Segar et al. (in press) found that midlife women who endorsed body shape motives for exercise were actually less physically active than those who exercised for other reasons. In an exercise intervention study with women ages 50 to 75, Shaw et al. (2000) found that, at baseline, percent of body fat was associated with poor physical self-concept and negative perceptions of physical appearance, but not associated with self-esteem. After the 9-month supervised exercise program, however, decrease in percent of body fat predicted improved perceptions of physical appearance, and the improvement was greatest in those women who had had lower self-esteem at baseline. In addition to its contribution to weight loss, exercise contributes to self-esteem and empowerment in a variety of ways. Building cardiovascular fitness and developing muscles results in physical strength, stamina, and increased energy. Enhanced fitness and strength contribute to independence and well-being as women find that they can do more things for themselves. Self-strengthening also reinforces self-efficacy, the belief that one is able to do what one wants to do (Chrisler & Lamont, 2002). These benefits of physical activity are important at any age, but perhaps even more so for midlife and older women.

McKinley (1999) recruited a sample of women college students (ages 17 to 22) and their mothers (ages 38 to 58) and surveyed them about their body image. The daughters had significantly higher scores on measures of body surveillance and body shame than their mothers did. There were no differences in body esteem between the groups even though the mothers weighed more and were less satisfied with their weight than the daughters were. Body esteem more strongly related to daughters' well-being than it did to mothers'. These data are interesting because they speak to the multidimensionality of both body image and self-esteem. Midlife women can be dissatisfied with their weight, yet not ashamed of it. They can feel good about themselves without experiencing the need to keep their physical appearance constantly in mind. McKinley (in press) surveyed the same women 10 years later and found that the mothers' (ages 48 to 68) body-esteem was relatively stable, even though their BMI had increased and they were exercising and dieting more. These data are consistent with some of the comments made by McFarland's midlife participants who said that they had learned to take care of their bodies and to judge them less harshly; they drew their self-esteem primarily from their accomplishments (McFarland, 1999).

McKinley (2004) also studied body esteem in a sample of 128 women ages 21 to 63, who were recruited from a list of subscribers to *Radiance*, a magazine aimed at heavy weight women. Among the questions she asked them were items about prejudice and discrimination against fat people and the need to seek social justice remedies. Those who endorsed the need for social change in attitudes toward fat people had higher body esteem and self-acceptance than did those who only endorsed the need for individuals to learn to accept themselves regardless of body size. In her in-depth interviews with 11 midlife Canadian women (ages 40 to 53) Banister (1999) heard comments from some women who actively resisted cultural beauty standards by labeling them as oppressive. The results of these two studies, combined with the findings of Tiggemann and Stevens (1999), suggest that midlife women's body esteem and self-esteem can be protected, at least to some extent, if they have a high consciousness of social justice issues. If cultural messages and societal strictures can be labeled as examples of sexism, ageism, or sizism, they can be more easily rejected. Perhaps midlife women would benefit from a revival of the consciousness-raising groups that were popular in the 1970s, which would provide an opportunity to discuss oppressive constraints on positive aging. Participants in such groups would no doubt come to the conclusion that the personal is still political.

Appearance Dissatisfaction

Research on the psychology of appearance has shown that qualities of the face are the most important determiners of attractiveness and that injury or illness that results in scarring or mutilation of the face and neck is the most difficult for people to accept (Bernstein, 1990). The Western beauty ideal demands a smooth, soft, and blemish-free face, but skin changes that occur with aging make this more and more difficult to achieve as the skin of the face and neck becomes drier and start to flake, loosen, and crease. Wrinkles or warts may appear on the face and "age" spot on the hands. In addition the hair may become thinner and grayer. The extent of these changes varies among individuals due to both genetic and environmental effects (Bernstein, 1990). Although the body image literature suggests that gradual changes (such as those caused by aging) are easier to adapt to than sudden changes (such as those caused by injuries) (Pruzinsky & Cash, 1990), such adaptation may be easier said than done for women, especially for those who have been closest to the beauty ideal, than it is for men due to the prevalent double standard of aging (Bernard, 1981; Sontag, 1979).

In a study of 268 adults (ages 18 to 80) from the southwestern United States, Harris (1994) found that signs of aging in both women and men were considered unattractive, but especially so in women. The participants expected women, more so than men, to take steps to conceal signs of aging as they appeared, and the women who participated in the study were significantly more likely than the men were to use (or to expect to use in the future) age concealment products or techniques. Harris' study is particularly interesting because, in addition to the attitudes survey, she asked participants to read scenarios in which midlife characters either did or did not make use of age concealment techniques. The participants judged those characters who tried to conceal their age more harshly than those who did not (i.e., they gave them higher ratings on such adjectives as "conceited," "foolish," "vain," "pathetic"), and this was true even for those participants who themselves practiced (or expected to practice) age concealment. McFarland's participants mentioned gray hair, wrinkles, double chins, and facial hair as signs of aging that they disliked (McFarland, 1999). Although some of the women were resigned to or philosophical about the changes, others worried that signs of aging could threaten their economic security by making it more difficult for them to get or keep a job, and they may be right about that given Harris' findings.

McLaren and Kuh (2004) reported high rates of body dissatisfaction among their sample of Canadian women in their 50s. When the researchers controlled for BMI, they found that body dissatisfaction was higher in women with higher socioeconomic status. Women with high socioeconomic status are likely to have the resources (e.g., time to exercise, money for cosmetics and surgery) necessary to allow them to approach the cultural beauty standard. Thus, we should not be surprised that they would worry more than other women about deviating further from the standard as they age. Yet, body dissatisfaction at midlife has been documented even in groups that are relatively protected from mainstream cultural beauty standards. Platte et al. (2000) surveyed a sample of Old Order Amish in rural Pennsylvania and found that older people (ages 45 to 66) were significantly more likely than younger people (ages 14 to 22) to report body dissatisfaction. Older women also tended to overestimate their body size.

However, not all studies show dissatisfaction with appearance at midlife. Deeks and McCabe (2001) reported that the older women in their sample (ages 35 to 65) were not more dissatisfied with their bodies overall than were the younger women, and Ross et al. (1989) reported that healthy older people (ages 62 to 79), although more conscious of their physical appearance than younger people (ages 17 to 28), actually evaluated their bodies more positively than the younger people did. In a survey of 678 women (ages 16 to 70) in the United Kingdom about their grooming rituals, Toerien et al. (2005) found that women over 50 were much less likely than younger women to remove their body hair, which suggests a willingness to deviate from the beauty standard. Davidson and McCabe (2005) reported that women in their 30s and 40s obtained higher body dissatisfaction scores and made more attempts at body concealment than did the younger and older women in their sample. The older women were less likely than the younger ones to engage in appearance comparisons, which suggests greater contentment with (or, at least, greater acceptance of) their bodies. The older women who were very concerned about other people's evaluations of their appearance were more depressed and anxious than the other women their age. In her interviews with 32 women ages 28 to 63, Giesen (1989) learned that single women were more likely than married women to believe that they were becoming more attractive and sexually appealing with age.

Donaldson (1994) reported that the participants in her sample (ages 40 to 59) had neutral to positive body image. They generally agreed that they were attractive to themselves and to others. Foerster (2001) conducted in-depth interviews with seven healthy women (ages 60 to 67), most of whom said that they were more accepting of themselves on a variety of dimensions than they had been earlier in life. The women referred to "making peace with" and "learning to like" their bodies (p. 42). Five of the women said that they were generally satisfied with their bodies, and three noted that their body image was better now than it had been when they were younger. When Foerster asked specifically what the women liked and disliked about their bodies, they mentioned disliking wrinkles, sagging skin, changes in their hair, knee problems, and extra weight around the abdomen; however, the majority said that they did not think about their looks very much. All said that they got positive appraisals of their appearance from others, especially their partners and friends. The women (ages 40 to 53) in Banister's study expressed similar mixed messages (Banister, 1999). Some spoke of being surprised to see reflections in mirrors or shop windows that look older than the women themselves feel. One recalled saying to herself: "My God, I look like my mother!" (p. 530). Another said: "If I look at myself, especially early in the morning [and see] all those wrinkles and saggy places, then I think, 'Gosh, I guess I am getting older!'" (p. 530). Yet another said: "... when I compare women my own age to women who are really young the young women's faces look so bland in a sense.... Life hasn't written its story on their faces" (p. 527).

Functional Dissatisfaction

Body image is as much about how the body functions and feels as it is about how the body appears to others, yet psychological researchers have focused much more on the body's ornamentality than its instrumentality. Although there are multidimensional measures of body image, in the research reviewed for this chapter the most common measures were the FRS, the Body Esteem Scale, and the Objectified Body Consciousness Scale, all of which are appearance-focused. Yet, we know that aging-related changes in functionality begin to be noticed in midlife, and thus may affect midlife women's body image in various ways. Changes that accompany aging or the onset and course of chronic illness may require the use of devices such as hearing aids, eyeglasses, pacemakers, or canes. These affect both one's appearance and bodily experience, as do surgical scars, limps or stiffness that result from injury or arthritis, hot flashes, imbalance, or side effects of medications (Hyman, 1987).

Changes in physical ability lead to restrictions in social and personal activities, which often result in lower self-esteem (Roberto & McGraw, 1991), as well as alterations in body image and self-concept. Osteoporosis is an example of a common disorder of older women that has physical, psychological, and social consequences. The fear of falling and fracturing a bone can cause women to restrict their activities (Roberto, 1990). Changes in body image have also been documented in women with rheumatoid arthritis and systemic lupus erythematosus (Cornwell & Schmitt, 1990). Body image disturbance was worse in the arthritis patients and more clearly related to the disease process, as the women reported that their major problems were due to mobility restriction. Body image disturbance in lupus patients was more closely related to the side effects of their medical regimen, and they reported that their major problems were fatigue and the need to avoid the sun. Cancer surgery, radiation treatments, and chemotherapy often cause fatigue, disfigurement, hair loss, and other physical changes that require psychological adjustment. Researchers have described body image issues in head and neck cancer (Bernstein, 1990), intestinal cancer (MacRitchie, 1980), breast cancer (e.g., Kriss & Kramer, 1986; Spencer et al., 1999), and uterine cancer (Schumacher, 1990). Allen and Wellard (2001) conducted in-depth interviews with four older women (ages 69 to 79) who recently had undergone cardiac surgery and now had large scars on their chests as a result of the sternotomy incision. The women reported that prior to the surgery they had been worried that they would be ashamed of the scars, that their partners would find them ugly, and that it would be difficult to find clothing that would conceal them. In retrospect, they were psychologically unaffected by the scars; health-related concerns were much more important to them.

Much of the psychosocial literature on breast cancer is informed by the assumption that mastectomy is psychologically devastating to women, much more so than any other type of amputation would be (Chrisler, 2001). This reflects the American cultural obsession with women's breasts and the belief that breasts are central to womanhood (Latteier, 1998). Thus, clinicians and American Cancer Society volunteers focus their efforts on body image issues, encourage women to apply makeup and wear feminine apparel after surgery, and urge women to have breast reconstruction surgery for mental health reasons (Kasper, 1995; Wilkinson & Kitzinger, 1993). However, in their review of the literature, Meyerowitz and Hart (1995) found that women with breast cancer do not report more distress than do women with other types of cancer or than do men with cancer. Women's main concerns are more likely to be survival, obtaining the best medical advice they can, worries about cancer recurrence, and questions about strength and physical ability after cancer treatment. Recent studies (Pecor, 2004; Spencer et al., 1999) of women who have been treated for breast cancer indicate that younger women exhibit more distress, more body dissatisfaction, and more sexual and partner-related concerns than do midlife and older women. There is some evidence that Black women are less distressed (Pecor, 2004) and Latinas have more body image disturbance (Spencer et al., 1999) than others after breast cancer surgery. Pecor (2004) theorized that older married women are more secure in their relationships and that older women in general, having experienced menopause, have learned to cope with bodily changes. Younger women are also, no doubt, more vulnerable to demands that they pursue the beauty ideal, and, before surgery, they had a better chance than midlife or older women of approaching it.

Menopause

The very fact of menopause requires an alteration in body image. Whether the cessation of the menstrual cycle is greeted with sadness, indifference, or relief it changes the way we think about our bodies (Chrisler & Ghiz, 1993). In addition, the physical signs (e.g., vaginal dryness, dry skin, thinning hair) that typically accompany menopause can affect body image. Vasomotor instability (e.g., hot flashes, night sweats) might make a woman feel that her once reliable body is out of control (Chrisler & Ghiz, 1993). How easily women adjust their body image in response to perimenopausal changes remains unclear, as most of the research on body image at midlife concerns weight and other aspects of appearance and body esteem.

Perimenopausal women in the United States have been depicted by the media as "diseased, hormone deficient, sexless, irritable, and depressed . . . and as passive victims of their changing hormones" (Golub, 1992, p. 215). This view has been encouraged by physicians and the pharmaceutical industry since the development in the 1960s of hormone replacement therapy (HRT; in earlier years—estrogen replacement therapy or ERT). Most books and magazine articles about menopause have examined the topic from a biomedical perspective, and, over the years, have suggested that HRT would keep women youthful, attractive, and both physically and mentally healthy (Chrisler et al., 1989; Gannon & Stevens, 1998). Although the promises of youth and beauty were debunked early on, beauty and health have since been conflated in our contemporary consumer culture, and television advertisements in the 1990s that featured supermodel Lauren Hutton (and other less known but attractive models) urging viewers to ask their doctors if HRT is right for them have no doubt perpetuated these old notions without naming them specifically. When the results of the Women's Health Initiative trials demonstrated that HRT is less beneficial (and for some women even harmful) than had been widely thought, many peri- and postmenopausal women stopped (or decided not to start) using HRT. However, it had been used primarily by well-educated, upper and upper-middle class women, those women who were, perhaps, closest to the cultural beauty standard and most interested in approaching it. In Deeks and McCabe's 2001 study, for example, only 18.4% of the peri- and postmenopausal participants reported current HRT use; another 3.9% had tried it but discontinued use.

Studies (Dillaway, 2005; Elson, 2002; Foerster, 2001; Maoz et al., 1970; Neugarten et al., 1968; Theisen et al., 1991) of women's attitudes toward menopause generally indicate ambivalence, or a mix of positive and negative attitudes. The realization that the fertility years are over is a stark reminder of aging for some women, and attitudes toward menopause are tied up with attitudes toward aging in general. The negative aspects that women have reported include the onset of aging, loss of fertility, loss of femininity, worries about emotional disturbance, worries about physical health, concerns about age-related changes rendering them unattractive or invisible, and a general sense that menopause has come too soon. Positive aspects of menopause that women have reported include no further need for contraception, no more menstrual periods, and a general sense of freedom from reproductive-related cares. It is interesting that younger women tend to have more negative attitudes toward menopause than older women do (Foerster, 2001; Neugarten et al., 1968). Foerster's participants (in their 60s) said that they had had negative expectations of the menopausal transition, but found that it was not so bad in retrospect. Some reported few, if any, physical symptoms; others reported "some symptoms or changes in appearance but were not bothered by them" (p. 42). The older women in Neugarten et al.'s classic study provide support for Margaret Mead's concept of "postmenopausal zest." They described postmenopausal women as "feeling better, more confident, calmer, and freer than before" (Golub, 1992, p. 216). In fact, most researchers report that women say that the worst thing about menopause is not knowing what to expect. It seems reasonable to predict that women with more positive (on balance) attitudes toward menopause would have an easier adjustment to menopause-related changes in body image, but there are, as yet, no data available to support or refute this hypothesis.

Midlife Body Image in the Context of Women's Lives

It is not surprising that when researchers ask women of any age how they feel about their bodies the women will respond with negative comments. The illusive beauty ideal and the cultural expectation of feminine modesty may combine to lead women to rate themselves toward the lower end of the scale when they evaluate their bodies, and this may be especially true on questionnaires that present women with a series of body parts. If women are asked "How satisfied are you with your thighs? With your nose? With your legs?", the demand is clearly for less than complete satisfaction. Even women who tend not to focus on their looks may think, "Well, my thighs are rather large, my nose could be cuter, etc." But if women in qualitative studies of midlife and aging routinely bring up body image concerns, that might be more persuasive evidence that body image issues are a problem.

Several recent studies suggest that body image issues are not near the top of the list of midlife women's concerns. Burns and Leonard (2005) conducted in-depth interviews with 60 midlife Australian women: 20 born between 1951 and 1956, 20 born between 1941 and 1946, and 20 born between 1931 and 1936. They began the interviews with an interesting strategy: the women were asked to think of their lives as a book and name the chapters. The chapter titles typically concerned turning points in life. It is interesting that the word "contentment" often appeared in the midlife chapter. The women saw midlife as a more satisfying time of life than most times in their past. It was described as a "break-out" time for women to try new things and leave behind old routines. Midlife represented more gains than losses and was considered to be a time of lowered stress due to children leaving home, retirement from jobs, and "living my own life at last" (p. 274). The women stressed the importance of self-actualization at midlife, and some actively questioned the traditional feminine gender role. Femininity might include beauty standards, but there was no mention of these in the article, which suggests that comments about bodily changes were not a common theme in the interviews.

Arnold (2005) surveyed 23 U.S. women ages 50 to 63, who were asked to write narratives in answer to a series of open-ended questions. Several of the questions could have provided space for women to raise body image concerns: "As you think about your life now, compared to your life in your 40s, in what ways (if any) has it changed?", "In what ways (if any) do you think you are different in the way you think and feel about things?", "Can you identify any specific life change events that have contributed to your current sense of self?", "As you think about the future, what are the things that concern or worry you the most?" (p. 637). Only two participants mentioned menopause as a life change event. The most prominent themes Arnold identified were "stepping out of the mold" (e.g., taking risks, dropping role demands, ignoring "shoulds"), "letting go" (e.g., of unrealistic expectations, of the need to acquire material goods), "walking in balance" (e.g., reordering priorities, seeking spiritual fulfillment, trusting oneself), "moving in new directions" (e.g., finding outlets for creative self-expression, finding new energy and zest for living, embarking on new careers), "redefining relationships" (e.g., moving away from stereotypical role boundaries, negotiating intimate relationships in more authentic ways), "freedom to be" (becoming more self-assured, making one's own choices), and "time as a precious commodity" (e.g., recognizing that life is finite and fragile, becoming more selective about how to spend one's time). None of the examples Arnold reported concern body image or body esteem explicitly, yet several themes are clearly related to a new (or increased) self-acceptance that might include the body. Learning to ignore shoulds, letting go of unrealistic expectations, finding new energy, making one's own choices, realizing that life is finite, and being more self-assured all should lead to greater acceptance and appreciation of the body one has and less time spent thinking about and pursuing an illusive beauty ideal.

The results of the Burns and Leonard (2005) and Arnold (2005) studies make an interesting contrast to Banister's in-depth interviews with 11 midlife Canadian women (ages 40 to 53) in which they were specifically asked about their changing bodies (Banister, 1999). Banister's participants provided the same mix of positive and negative comments that have been reported in the attitudes toward menopause studies. The women commented that they've gained weight, that the menopausal body "is unfamiliar again" (p. 527), that "things are falling" (p. 526), and that they feel "different" (p. 529). They spoke about their growing awareness that life is finite, which Banister connected to their "loss of youthful appearance, loss of youthful energy, and loss of fertility" (p. 529). Yet the comments of the individual women often showed more body acceptance than the general themes might suggest. One said: "Now in some ways I am influenced by our culture ... in other ways I'm pretty happy with my body" (p. 526). Another said: "There's a bit more weight here and there, but I feel that my body looks good for being 52" (p. 526). One of the main themes in the interviews was "caring for self," which referred to physical, psychological, and spiritual self-care. The women said that they were learning to question social norms and cultural expectations, to put their own needs first, to put time and effort into taking care of their bodies, and to reflect on being a part of nature. These comments are similar to those made by Arnold's and Burns and Leonard's participants, and, again, they indicate a blend of bodily acceptance and self-redefinition that suggests that the women are adjusting well to changes in their body image.

Authenticity

The comments made by the participants in the qualitative studies reviewed above suggest a midlife striving for authenticity. Some reasons why women value breaking out, redefinition of self, and the freedom "to be" are that the growth in wisdom and self-confidence, the loosening of role demands (e.g., grown children, retirement), and, yes, even the invisibility associated with midlife allow for greater choice and flexibility in how one spends one's time and energy. The realization that life is finite, which accompanies midlife and is especially associated with menopause and diagnoses of chronic illness, has the benefit of focusing the mind on a reorganization of priorities that allows women to put their own needs first and decide how to live their own lives. A conscious reorganization provides the perfect opportunity for midlife women to decide to take care of their bodies (e.g., by feeding them properly, allowing adequate time for rest, scheduling a massage) rather than to torment their bodies (e.g., by chronic dieting, compulsive exercise, scheduling a facelift) in an increasingly hopeless attempt to approach the beauty ideal.

Beauty rituals are time-consuming activities. Jokes about how long women take to get ready to go out are based on the many tasks that women do (and men do not) when they are getting dressed, and with age these rituals are more demanding (Saltzberg & Chrisler, 1995). It takes time to pluck eyebrows, shave legs, manicure nails, apply makeup, and arrange hair. Women's clothing is more complicated than men's (especially at midlife when body shape changes make "foundation garments" necessary if women wish to wear fashionable clothes). Although all women know that the "transformation from female to feminine is artificial" (Chapkis, 1986, p. 5), we conspire to hide the amount of time and effort it takes, perhaps out of fear that other women do not need as much time as we do to appear beautiful (Saltzberg & Chrisler, 1995). To be artificial, of course, is to be inauthentic. To choose to be authentic is to gain time (and money!) for more important or pleasurable pursuits.

Yet to turn one's back on the beauty ideal after years of pursuing it is easier said than done. Cultural messages that to "age gracefully" is to "age successfully" (Calasanti et al., 2006) merge with messages that promote the importance of beauty and thinness for women of all ages to encourage midlife women to "pass" as young for as long as they can (Ostenson, 2004). Passing, whether it refers to light-skinned African Americans "allowing" others to assume they are "White" or lesbians wearing mainstream attire and keeping quiet about their personal lives so that others will assume they are heterosexual, can involve one-time, temporary acts (e.g., lying about one's age on a job application, getting a botox injection) or an act or series of acts with long-term implications (e.g., regularly coloring one's gray hair, getting a facelift). Regardless of whether passing is applauded ("you look so young for your age!") or denigrated (e.g., people who conceal signs of aging are pathetic; Harris, 1994), it is an inauthentic act, a denial of a person's identity, experience, and maturity (Ostenson, 2004). A preoccupation with passing will not help women to experience the striving for authenticity reported by the midlife women in the qualitative studies discussed above; in fact, it might hinder their ability to relax into living their own lives.

Cultural messages about beauty and femininity overlap, as the former is generally considered to be a prerequisite for the latter. Therefore, feminine women may place more emphasis on beauty (Gillen & Lefkowitz, in press) and may have a harder time adjusting to bodily changes at midlife. Pliner et al. (1990) reported a correlation between high femininity scores and greater appearance orientation in girls and women ages 10 to 79. Pecor (2004) found that women with higher femininity scores reported more distress and poorer psychosocial adjustment after breast cancer surgery than did women who were classified as masculine or androgynous, and Mahalik et al. (2005) included subscales on "thinness" and "investment in appearance" in their new Conformity to Feminine Norms Inventory. Cultural messages about femininity also encourage inauthenticity in interpersonal relationships (e.g., women should fake orgasms and express interest in whatever topics or hobbies interest their partners), and Gillen and Lefkowitz (in press) found that women college students who were less instrumental and more inauthentic in their relationships also had more negative attitudes toward their bodies.

It would be interesting to know whether high femininity predicts more body image concerns at midlife, and there is some evidence to support this notion. For example, lesbians (Donaldson, 1994) and feminists (Tiggemann & Stevens, 1999) express less weight concern that other women do, and they are also probably more likely than heterosexual nonfeminists to question traditional gender roles and gendered expectations. Perhaps Black women are less likely to consider themselves overweight (Stevens et al., 1994) and less distressed after breast cancer treatment (Pecor, 2004) because Black women are more likely than White women to behave androgynously. Latinas, on the other hand, are generally thought to be more traditional in their gender role attitudes, and that might account for part of the reason why they have been shown to be more distressed than Black and White women after breast cancer treatment (Spencer et al., 1999). In addition, participants in the qualitative studies (Arnold, 2005; Burns & Leonard, 2005) mentioned that as they aged they increasingly questioned (and resisted) the traditional feminine gender role.

Conclusion

Much remains to be learned about body image issues and adjustments of women over 50. What little we know is concentrated on weight and appearance; much less work has been done on functional changes and on the menopausal transition. There are hints that women who are in better health, who are in stable long-term relationships and/or are sexually active, and who are more nontraditional in their gender role orientation will have a more positive body image at midlife. However, these relations need to be tested directly.

Furthermore, the research on midlife and older women rarely includes longitudinal data or samples large enough to contrast cohorts with each other. In most cases there is no way to know if women in their 50s differ from women in their 40s, 60s, and 70s. It is also impossible at this point to tell whether data about women in their 50s today would differ from data about women who were in their 50s 20 years ago or those who will be in their 50s 20 years from now. Women who are currently in their 50s and 60s were impacted strongly by the Women's Liberation Movement, and, therefore, one might expect them to be less traditional in their attitudes, more comfortable with themselves, and more willing to resist cultural messages that they should take steps to conceal signs of aging and pass as younger than they are. One can only wonder about how women in their 20s and 30s today, the so-called postfeminist generation, will cope with aging. They came of age in a time of hyperconsumerism, where there is a "cure" for almost everything and where women are expected to be both beautiful and high achieving. Only time will tell how they will confront signs of aging.

It is interesting that the quantitative studies of body esteem and appearance concerns yield different information than do qualitative studies that address midlife and aging more generally. Perhaps what we need are mixed method studies in which both standardized scales and interviews or focus groups are used. This might help us to understand how focused women are on bodily changes and concerns and, if negative body image is an important issue for them, to provide clues about how to design appropriate interventions.

Like most things in life, aging is neither all good nor all bad. Experience, maturation, development, lifecycle transitions, and even invisibility are both benefits and challenges. Midlife, with its focus on finding balance and reorganizing priorities, can be the perfect time to stop fighting our bodies and learn to appreciate them. Our stretch marks, scars, gray hairs, and extra pounds are proof of who we are and what we've been through to get where we are. Let us embrace the bodily changes we like as well as those we do not, resist the impulse to alter ourselves in inauthentic ways, and take good and gentle care of ourselves so that our bodies will last long enough for us to gain even more wisdom and experience. Let us not waste the precious time we have left in trying to be what we are not.

References

Alderson, B.W. (1991, March). *An Overview of Emotional Issues Faced by Women Over 50*. Paper presented at the meeting of the Association for Women in Psychology, Hartford, CT.

Allen, K.E., and Wellard, S.J. (2001). Older women's experiences with sternotomy. *International Journal of Nursing Practice, 7*, 274–279.

Arnold, E. (2005). A voice of their own: Women moving into their fifties. *Health Care for Women International, 26*, 630–651.

Banister, E.M. (1999). Women's midlife experiences of their changing bodies. *Qualitative Health Research, 9*, 520–537.

Bernard, J. (1981). *The Female World.* New York: Free Press.
Bernstein, N.R. (1990). Objective bodily damage: Disfigurement and dignity. In T.F. Cash and T. Pruzinsky (Eds.), *Body Images: Development, Deviance, and Change* (pp. 131–169). New York: Guilford.
Burns, A., and Leonard, R. (2005). Chapters of our lives: Life narratives of midlife and older Australian women. *Sex Roles, 52*, 269–277.
Calasanti, T., Sleven, K.F., and King, N. (2006). Ageism and feminism: From "et cetera" to center. *NWSA Journal, 18*, 13–30.
Chapkis, W. (1986). *Beauty Secrets: Women and the Politics of Appearance.* Boston: South End Press.
Chrisler, J.C. (2001). Gendered bodies and physical health. In R.K. Unger (Ed.), *Handbook of the Psychology of Women and Gender* (pp. 289–302). New York: Wiley.
Chrisler, J.C., and Ghiz, L. (1993). Body image issues of older women. *Women & Therapy, 14*(1/2), 67–75.
Chrisler, J.C., and Lamont, J.M. (2002). Can exercise contribute to the goals of feminist therapy? *Women & Therapy, 25*(2), 9–22.
Chrisler, J.C., Torrey, J.W., and Matthes, M. (1989, June). *Brittle Bones and Sagging Breasts, Loss of Femininity and Loss of Sanity: The Media Describe the Menopause.* Paper presented at the meeting of the Society for Menstrual Cycle Research, Salt Lake City.
Cornwell, C.J., and Schmitt, M.H. (1990). Perceived health status, self-esteem, and body image in women with rheumatoid arthritis or systemic lupus erythematosus. *Research in Nursing and Health, 13*, 99–107.
Davidson, T.E., and McCabe, M.P. (2005). Relationships between men's and women's body image and their psychological, social, and sexual functioning. *Sex Roles, 52*, 463–475.
Davis, D.M. (1990). Portrayals of women in prime-time network television: Some demographic characteristics. *Sex Roles, 23*, 35–332.
Deeks, A.A., and McCabe, M.P. (2001). Menopausal stage and age and perceptions of body image. *Psychology and Health, 16*, 367–379.
Dillaway, H.E. (2002). (Un)Changing menopausal bodies: How women think and act in the face of a reproductive transition and gendered beauty ideals. *Sex Roles, 53*, 1–17.
Donaldson, G.A. (1994). *Body Image in Women at Midlife.* Unpublished doctoral dissertation, Boston College.
Elson, J. (2002). Menarche, menstruation, and gender identity: Retrospective accounts from women who have undergone premenopausal hysterectomy. *Sex Roles, 46*, 37–48.
Fallon, A.E., and Rozin, P. (1985). Sex differences in perceptions of desirable body shape. *Journal of Abnormal Psychology, 94*, 102–105.
Foerster, G. (2001). *The Relationship between Body Image and Sexuality for Women in their Sixties: A Qualitative Study.* Unpublished doctoral dissertation, California School of Professional Psychology.
Fooken, I. (1994). Sexuality in the later years: The impact of health and body image in a sample of older women. *Patient Education and Counseling, 23*, 227–233.
Franks, V., and Fodor, I. (Guest Eds.). (1990). Women at midlife and beyond [special issue]. *Psychology of Women Quarterly, 14*(4).
Freedman, R. (1986). *Beauty Bound.* Lexington, MA: D.C. Heath.
Ganon, L., and Stevens, J. (1998). Portraits of menopause in the media. *Women & Health, 27*(3), 1–15.
Gerbner, G., Gross, L., Signorielli, N., and Morgan, M. (1980). Aging with television: Images on television drama and conceptions of social reality. *Journal of Communication, 30*, 37–47.

Gerike, A.E. (1990). On gray hair and oppressed brains. *Journal of Women & Aging, 1*(1/2/3), 35–46.

Giesen, C.B. (1989). Aging and attractiveness: Marriage makes a difference. *International Journal of Aging and Human Development, 29*, 83–94.

Gillen, M.M., and Lefkowitz, E.S. (in press). Gender role development and body mage among male and female first year college students. *Sex Roles.*

Glascock, J. (2001). Gender roles on prime-time network television: Demographics and behaviors. *Journal of Broadcasting and Electronic Media, 45*, 656–669.

Golub, S. (1992). *Periods: From Menarche to Menopause.* Newbury Park, CA: Sage.

Greenspan, M. (1983). *A New Approach to Women and Therapy.* New York: McGraw-Hill.

Gupta, M.A., and Schork, N.J. (1993). Aging-related concerns and body image: Possible future implications for eating disorders. *International Journal of Eating Disorders, 14*, 481–486.

Harris, M.B. (1994). Growing old gracefully: Age concealment and gender. *Journal of Gerontology, 49*, P149–P158.

Hays, K.F. (1999). *Working it Out: Using Exercise in Psychotherapy.* Washington, DC: American psychological Association.

Hyman, J. (1987). Who needs cosmetic surgery? Reassessing our looks and our lives. In Boston Women's Health Book Collective (Eds.), *Our Bodies, Ourselves: Growing Older* (pp. 37–45). New York: Simon & Schuster.

Kasper, A.S. (1995). The social construction of breast loss and reconstruction. *Women's Health, 1*, 197–219.

Kriss, R.T., and Kramer, H.C. (1986). Efficacy of group therapy for problems with post-mastectomy self-perception, body image, and sexuality. *Journal of Sex Research, 22*, 438–451.

Lamb, C.S., Jackson, L.A., Cassiday, P.B., and Priest, D.J. (1993). Body figure preferences of men and women: A comparison of two generations. *Sex Roles, 28*, 345–358.

Latteier, C. (1998). *Breasts: The Women's Perspective on an American Obsession.* New York: Harrington Park Press.

Lauzen, M.M., and Dozier, D.M. (2995). Maintaining the double standard: Portrayals of age and gender in popular films. *Sex Roles, 52*, 437–446.

Lewis, D.M., and Cachelin, F.M. (2001). Body image, body dissatisfaction, and eating attitudes in midlife and elderly women. *Eating Disorders, 9*, 29–39.

MacRitchie, K.J. (1980). Prenatal nutrition outside the hospital: Psychosocial styles of adaptation. *Canadian Journal of Psychiatry, 25*, 308–313.

Mahalik, J.R., Morray, E.B., Coonerty-Femiano, A., Ludlow, L.H., Slattery, S.M., and Smiler, A. (2005). Development of the Conformity to Feminine Norms Inventory. *Sex Roles, 52*, 417–435.

Markey, C.N., Markey, P.M., and Birch, L.L. (2004). Understanding women's body satisfaction: The role of husbands. *Sex Roles, 51*, 209–216.

Maoz, B., Dowty, N., Antonovsky, A., and Wijsenbeek, H. (1970). Female attitudes to menopause. *Social Psychiatry, 5*, 35–40.

McFarland, M.B. (1999). *A Descriptive Study of Body Dysphoria and Body Image in Midlife Women.* Unpublished doctoral dissertation, University of North Dakota.

McKinley, N.M. (1999). Women and objectified body consciousness: Mothers' and daughters' body experience in cultural, developmental, and familial context. *Developmental Psychology, 35*, 760–769.

McKinley, N.M. (2004). Resisting body dissatisfaction: Fat women who endorse fat acceptance. *Body Image, 1*, 213–219.

McKinley, N.M. (2006). The developmental and cultural contexts of objectified body consciousness: A longitudinal analysis of two cohorts of women. *Developmental Psychology, 42*, 679–687.

McLaren, L., and Kuh, D. (2004). Body dissatisfaction in midlife women. *Journal of Women & Aging, 16*(1/2), 35–54.

Meyerowitz, B.E., and Hart, S. (1995). Women and cancer: Have assumptions about women limited our research agenda? In A.L. Stanton and S.J. Gallant (Eds.), *Psychology of Women's Health: Progress and Challenges in Research and Applications* (pp. 51–84). Washington, DC: American psychological Association.

Miller, D.J. (2001). Weight satisfaction among Black and White couples: The role of perceptions. *Eating Disorders, 9*, 41–47.

Nett, E.M. (1991). Is there life after fifty? Images of middle age for women in *Chatelaine* magazine. *Journal of Women & Aging, 3*(1), 93–115.

Neugarten, B.L., Wood, V., Kraines, R.J., and Loomis, B. (1968). Women's attitudes toward menopause. In B.L. Neugarten (Ed.), Middle age and aging (pp. 195–200). Chicago: University of Chicago Press.

O'Brien, J. (1980, April 24). Mirror, mirror: Why me? *Nursing Mirror*, pp. 36–37.

Ostenson, R. (2004). Who's in and who's out: The results of oppression. In J.C. Chrisler, C. Golden, and P.D. Rozee (Eds.), *Lectures on the Psychology of Women* (3rd ed., pp. 16–26). Boston: McGraw-Hill.

Pecor, M.J. (2004). *The Impact of Breast Cancer on Body Image in Ethnically Diverse Women*. Unpublished doctoral dissertation, Auburn University.

Pettus, M. (2001). Kudos for me: Self-esteem. In J.J. Robert-McComb (Ed.), *Eating Disorders in Women and Children: Prevention, Stress Management, and Treatment* (pp. 283–290). Boca Raton, FL: CRC Press.

Piercy, M. (2006). I met a woman who wasn't there. *NWSA Journal, 18*, 1–2.

Platte, P., Zelton, J.F., and Stunkard, A.J. (2000). Body image in the Old Order Amish: A people separate from "the world." *International Journal of Eating Disorders, 28*, 408–414.

Pliner, P., Chaiken, S., and Flett, G.L. (1990). Gender differences in concern with body weight and physical appearance over the lifespan. *Personality and Social Psychology Bulletin, 16*, 263–273.

Pruzinsky, T., and Cash, T.F. (1990). Integrative themes in body image development, deviance, and change. In T.F. Cash and T. Pruzinsky (Eds.), *Body Images: Development, Deviance, and Change* (pp. 337–349). New York: Guilford.

Rackley, J.V., Warren, S.A., & Bird, G.W. (1988). Determinants of body image in women at midlife. *Psychological Reports, 62*, 9–10.

Roberto, K.A. (1990). Adjusting to chronic disease: The osteoporotic woman. *Journal of Women & Aging, 2*(1), 33–47.

Roberto, K.A., and McGraw, S. (1991). Self-perceptions of older women with osteoporosis. *Journal of Women & Aging, 3*(1), 59–70.

Rodin, J., Silberstein, L., and Striegel-Moore, R. (1984). Women and weight: A normative discontent. In T. Sonderegger (Ed.), *Nebraska Symposium on Motivation* (pp. 267–304). Lincoln, NE: University of Nebraska Press.

Ross, M.J., Tait, R.C., Grossberg, G.T., Hamdal, P.J., Brandeberry, L., and Nakra, R. (1989). Age differences in body consciousness. *Journal of Gerontology, 44*, P23–P24.

Rozin, P., and Fallon, A. (1988). Body image, attitudes toward weight, and misperceptions of figure preferences of the opposite sex: A comparison of men and women in two generations. *Journal of Abnormal Psychology, 97*, 342–345.

Saltzberg, E.A., and Chrisler, J.C. (1995). Beauty is the beast: Psychological effects of the pursuit of the perfect female body. In J. Freeman (Ed.), *Women: A Feminist Perspective* (5th ed., pp. 306–315). Mountain View, CA: Mayfield.

Schumacher, D. (1990). Hidden death: The sexual effects of hysterectomy. *Journal of Women & Aging, 2*(2), 49–66.

Segar, M., Spruijt-Metz, D., and Nolen-Hoeksema, S. (2006). Go figure? Body shape motives are associated with decreased physical activity participation among midlife women. *Sex Roles, 54*, 175–187.

Shaw, J.M., Ebbeck, V., and Snow, C.M. (2000). Body composition and physical self-concept in older women. *Journal of Women & Aging, 12*(3/4), 59–75.

Sontag, S. (1979). The double standard of aging. In J.H. Williams (Ed.), *Psychology of Women: Selected Readings* (pp. 462–478). New York: W.W. Norton.

Spencer, S.M., Lehman, J.M., Wynings, C., Arena, P., Carver, C.S., Antoni, M.H., Derhagopian, R.P., Ironson, G., and Love, N. (1999). Concerns about breast cancer and relations to psychosocial well-being in a multiethnic sample of early-stage patients. *Health Psychology, 18*, 159–168.

Stevens, J., Kumanyika, S.K., and Keil, J.E. (1994). Attitudes toward body size and dieting: Differences between elderly Black and White women. *American Journal of Public Health, 84*, 1322–1325.

Stokes, R., and Frederick-Recascino, C. (2003). Women's perceived body image: Relations with personal happiness. *Journal of Women & Aging, 15*(1), 17–29.

Theisen, C.X., Mansfield, P.K., Voda, A.M., and Seery, B. (1991, June). *Predictors of Attitudes Toward Menopause among Midlife Women*. Paper presented at the meeting of the Society for Menstrual Cycle Research, Seattle.

Tiggemann, M., and Stevens, C. (1999). Weight concern across the life-span: Relationship to self-esteem and feminist identity. *International Journal of Eating Disorders, 26*, 103–106.

Toerien, M., Wilkinson, S., and Choi, P.Y.L. (2005). Body hair removal: The 'mundane' production of normative femininity. *Sex Roles, 52*, 399–406.

Vernon, J.A., Williams, J.A. Jr., Phillips, T., and Wilson, J. (1991). Media stereotyping: A comparison of the way elderly women and men are portrayed on prime-time television. *Journal of Women & Aging, 2*(4), 55–68.

Voda, A.M., Christy, N.S., and Morgan, J.M. (1991). Body composition changes in menopausal women. *Women & Therapy, 11*(2), 71–96.

White, J.W. (2005). *Psychology of Women Quarterly*, 2000–2004. *Psychology of Women Quarterly, 29*, 107–109.

Wilcox, S.J. (1996). *Sex and Age Differences in Body Attitudes Across the Adult Life-Span*. Unpublished doctoral dissertation, Washington University.

Wilkinson, S., and Kitzinger, C. (1993). Whose breast is it anyway? A feminist consideration of advice and treatment for breast cancer. *Women's Studies International Forum, 16*, 229–238.

Wolf, N. (1991). *The Beauty Myth: How Images of Beauty are Used Against Women*. New York: Morrow.

Young, C.M., Blondin, J., Tensuan, R., and Fryer, J.H. (1963). Body composition studies of older women, 30–70 years of age. *Annals of the New York Academy of Sciences, 110*, 589–607.

2
Women and Sex at Midlife: Desire, Dysfunction, and Diversity

Maureen C. McHugh

Are women likely to experience more sexual and relationship satisfaction in midlife than in earlier periods of their lives? Which women are, and why? Does a woman experience heterosexual partner sex more positively when she is no longer responsible for birth control or parenting? In what ways, if any, do the sexual relations of aging lesbians improve over time? Are women who are autoerotic more likely to be in touch with their own sexual desire than women who are dependent on partners for sexual arousal and activity? Is sexual authenticity an important component in the positive sexual response of older women? These are examples of possible research (and personal) questions that cannot be answered at this point. Researchers have not typically investigated the possible positive sexual feelings and experiences of women at midlife. Rather, the literature has focused almost exclusively on the possible declines in sexual activity and desire allegedly experienced by women as a result of declining hormones. The research on women and sexuality at midlife both reflects and reifies the negative cultural views and disease-oriented medical perspectives on aging that are present today in many societies. The current research is reviewed acknowledging the degree to which limited perspectives on women's sexuality has limited our understanding of the sexuality of women at midlife and beyond.

The idea that women's sexuality declines at midlife, adversely affected by menopause, is widely held by the general public and by many professionals. Middle age is a developmental stage marked by changes at multiple levels, and many women report changes in their intimate relationships, as well as in sexual interest, responsiveness, and behavior. Menopause, the cessation of the menstrual cycle and the declining levels of estrogen, is only one aspect of the changes that occur in middle-aged women's lives. Menopause occurs during the 40s and 50s when other aging processes also occur, when the woman's roles and family structures are often changing, when her partner, if she has one, is also aging, and when she is viewed differently than younger women in her culture and society. Thus, there are many potential influences on women's intimate relationships and sexual responses at midlife. A substantial amount of the research on women's sexuality in midlife and beyond has focused on the role of menopause and has been conducted from within the medical or biological position. Research conducted from the biomedical perspective emphasizes the relationship between declining hormones and declines in women's sexual desire, activity, and satisfaction. A medical perspective on women's sexuality has been increasingly emphasized, as researchers investigate pharmaceutical "solutions" to women's sexual "problems."

Critics (e.g., Koch et al., 2005; Wood et al., in press) have pointed out that the dominant perspective is based on a medical or physiological model of the human sexual response cycle and upon the assumption that sexual desire is the component in that cycle that is most influenced by hormonal factors. Although many have linked changes in women's sexual responsiveness at midlife to declining hormones, an increasing number of researchers have criticized the biomedical perspective on menopause and declining sexual response (e.g., Koch et al., 2005; Morokoff, 1988; Tiefer, 1995; Voda & George, 1986). Existing models tend to emphasize the physiological aspects of desire and minimize the importance of contextual factors (Basson, 2002; Kaschak & Tiefer, 2001; Wood et al., in press). In contrast, the feminist and social interpretive perspectives emphasize the ways in which sexuality is influenced by other factors including relationship quality and sociohistorical context (Koch et al., 2005). The research on the sexual desire of women in their 50s is reviewed here from a feminist perspective.

To suggest that the sexuality of women at midlife is a function of menopause homogenizes women. Even the documented biological effects of menopause are experienced in a particular sociohistorical context, and women's experience of them is by no means homogenous. Women's understanding of both menopause and sexuality impacts their constructions of their own sexual experiences as satisfying or problematic. In this chapter I emphasize the contextual factors that influence women's constructions of and experiences of menopause and sexuality at midlife. My review also emphasizes the variability in women's sexuality in midlife and beyond and the possibilities presented by women's accounts of their own lives.

Declining Hormones and Women's Sexuality

Physical Effects of Menopause

Sexual enjoyment may be impacted by the physical changes that occur as estrogen levels decline. One of the main effects of reduced estrogen levels is a reduction in vaginal lubrication. After menopause, it often takes longer to become moist during sexual arousal. However, it is important to realize that vaginal dryness at this, or any, age may simply be an indication that the woman is not ready for intercourse. With insufficient lubrication, penetration may be uncomfortable or painful, and intercourse may lead to irritation or infection (Boston Women's Health Book Collective, 2005). During the menopausal transition, the vaginal walls generally become thinner, drier, and less flexible, and they may be vulnerable to tears and cracks. Some medications, such as antihistamines, may contribute to vaginal dryness, and soaps, sprays, and perfumed toilet paper can irritate the vulva (Boston Women's Health Book Collective, 2005). As vaginal tissue becomes thinner, penetration may result in bleeding. Vaginal dryness and hot flashes, two conditions that occur along with declining estrogen, have been linked to declining sexual responsiveness (McCoy et al., 1985).

Both mental and physical health can impact sexual functioning. As women age, various health conditions may impact their sexual response. Menopause-related problems, such as heavy bleeding or urinary leaking, can adversely impact women's sexual interest and experience. Additional physical problems that can impact sexual interactions were outlined by Diokno et al. (1990) based on research with individuals 60 years of age or older: decreased mobility, incontinence, use of sedatives, and a history of heart attacks. Other health problems experienced as a result of aging, such as diabetes or high blood pressure, can also affect lovemaking or sexual interest. Women may feel less sexual as a result of chronic or acute illnesses due to pain or fatigue. Arthritic disease may hamper sexual activity. In both research and clinical practice it is important to consider the impact of specific health problems rather than simply attributing women's problems or symptoms to aging or menopause (Boston Women's Health Book Collective, 2005).

Women's Sexual Problems at Midlife and Beyond

The incidence of sexual problems is high among women of all ages (Leiblum & Pervin, 1980), and women report increased sexual problems during the menopausal years (Bachmann et al., 1989; Leiblum, 1990). When women's sexual problems are defined as discontent or dissatisfaction with any emotional, physical, or relational aspect of sexual experience, many women report that they have a "problem" (McHugh, in press). In a national survey of more than 2500 women, 99% of women reported experiencing at least one of the 23 sexual problems listed (Ellison, 2001). Not only are there many problems, but there are many different causes and contributing factors for women's sexual problems (McHugh, in press; Williams, 2001).

Cole (1988) reported on clinical interviews with 100 women who were clients at a Menopause Clinic; 85 of the 100 women reported at least one sexual problem. Common problems included: vaginal dryness, loss of clitoral sensation, and decreased frequency of sex. Some of the reports from women suggest a loss of desire. For example, women reported a loss of sex drive and interest, loss of enjoyment, inability to become aroused, and lack of responsiveness. Some women reported problems with masturbation as well as with partner sex. Similarly, Leiblum (1990) reported that menopausal women in her study reported a decline in interest and desire and problems attaining orgasm. Some women in each study reported the experience of dyspareunia, that is, painful intercourse. The anticipation of painful intercourse may interfere with relaxation and inhibit desire. In the research reported by Diokno et al. (1990), 40% of the men said that they were having erectile problems, and 9 to 10% of men and women said that they were having difficulty with intercourse. Diokno et al. also found that sexual activity decreases with age. In their sample of senior (60+) individuals, 66% of men, but only 32% of women, reported that they were sexually active. In an early study conducted by the Center for the Study of Aging at Duke University (Pfeiffer et al., 1972) declines in sexual responsiveness were reported by both men and women. In that large study of biologically and socially advantaged individuals born before 1900, respondents indicated a substantial decline in sexual interest and activity; 6% of the men and 33% of the women reported not being interested in sex, and 12% of the men and 40% of the women reported no longer engaging in sex.

Declines in Women's Sexual Desire

A common conclusion is that women experience a decrease in sexual desire as a result of menopausal declines in hormones. For example, McCoy and Davidson (1985) investigated changes in sexual interest and coital frequency of a small group of married women enrolled in a longitudinal study. The sample included women who were premenopausal, perimenopausal, and menopausal. Participants kept daily records of menstrual and coital events, gave regular blood samples, and were interviewed at 4-month intervals until they were menopausal. At each interview, participants rated their sexual experience, their symptoms, and their sexual responsiveness for the past 30 days. The data indicate that menopause impacted lubrication and that coital frequency declined with menopause. The data also indicate that sexual interest, as indicated by reported sexual thoughts or fantasies, decreased with menopause; 14 of 16 participants reported such a decrease. In a related study McCoy et al. (1985) studied a sample of White, middle-class, and highly educated, middle-aged, perimenopausal women. The respondents reported changes in sexual response as the fourth most common change they had experienced. Almost one-half of the respondents reported that their current sexual response seemed "different." Experiencing less desire was the most commonly reported change (54%), but 15% reported experiencing more desire. Approximately one-quarter of the respondents reported each of the following changes: more enjoyment with a partner, less enjoyment with a partner, and more difficulty experiencing orgasm. Based on regression analyses, the authors reported that marital status and vaginal dryness predicted changes in sexual desire and sexual enjoyment, and age was also a significant predictor of changes in sexual enjoyment. Menopausal status, however, did not predict any of the dependent variables of sexual desire, sexual enjoyment, or experience of orgasm. Rather than emphasizing the physiological or hormonal aspects of aging, the authors argued for the development of multiple and more integrated approaches to the study of women's sexuality across the lifespan.

Dennerstein et al. (1999, 2001) used a longitudinal analysis and structural equation modeling to disentangle the effects of change in menopausal status from the effects of age on sexuality. Their longitudinal study (Dennerstein et al., 2001) began in 1991 with a random sample of 2000 Australian women aged 45 to 55 years. Eight years later, the sexuality responses of women who had passed through the menopausal transition were compared to those of women who remained premenopausal and women who were postmenopausal for the same length of time. The menopausal group reported a significant overall decline in sexual functioning, especially in sexual responsivity. During this phase, the partner's problems with sexual performance increased significantly, and women's positive feelings for the partner declined significantly. Frequency of sexual activity and sexual desire decreased most in the menopausal phase. The longitudinal study confirms the earlier structural equation model finding that both age and menopausal status contribute to declines in women's sexual functioning. Although both analyses confirmed the effects of aging and menopause, the authors stressed that women's relationships with their partners had a particularly powerful effect on women's sexual desire, a fact that is often lost in discussions of sexuality and aging.

To challenge the biomedical model, Mansfield et al. (2000) asked a sample of 505 White, married, middle-aged women about their sexual responses and their own understanding of any changes. The women were recruited from the Tremin Trust Research Program and from the 1963 graduating class of Douglass College. Postmenopausal hormone users were not included. Forty percent of the respondents indicated some change in their sexual response. The changes were primarily decrements in desire, arousal, enjoyment, and/or decreases in the frequency of sex and orgasm. The majority of those who reported changes reported: desiring sex less (64%), having sex less often (57%), desiring more nongenital touching (55%), and finding arousal more difficult (53%). The women attributed changes involving a decline in their response to physical and emotional changes as related to menopause, whereas increases in responsiveness were attributed to changing life circumstances.

Note that the researchers who reported declining levels of sexual activity and/or desire in midlife did not report that this was the case for all of the women in their samples. Variability, including the fact that some women experience increases in desire, can be found in the literature (Dennerstein et al., 2003; Hallstrom, 1977; Hallstrom & Samuelson, 1990; Mansfield et al., 1998; McCoy & Davidson, 1985), and not all researchers have reported a significant decline in women's sexual response during midlife. Increases in sexual response or a lack of substantive changes have been reported (Bachmann et al., 1989; Dennerstein et al., 1997). For example, no significant changes in pre- or postmenopausal sexual responses of middle aged women were reported by the women in Cutler and colleagues' study (Cutler et al., 1987). Women aged 33 to 56 were recruited from the Bay area for a study of menopause and responded to a 31 item questionnaire that assessed their sexual desire, sexual response, and sexual satisfaction in relation to steroid levels in the perimenopausal period (Cutler et al., 1987). Questions about frequency of masturbation, intercourse, sexual thoughts, and arousal, and items that concerned satisfaction, pleasure, orgasm, distress, dysfunction, and dyspareunia were examined in relation to changes related to the menstrual cycle. Women did not report a decline in arousability; most reported that sexual arousal occurred in every sexual episode. The overwhelming majority (86%) did not experience deficits in lubrication, and dyspareunia was rarely encountered. No recent change was perceived by the respondents in frequency of fantasies. However, women with low estradiol levels did report a decline in frequency of intercourse.

Similarly, a longitudinal study of married women living in a Swedish city showed evidence for stability of sexual desire through the premenopausal period (Hallstrom

& Samuelson, 1990). The research involved data collected from a representative sample of 800 middle-aged, married women (from cohorts born in 1914, 1918, 1922, and 1930) who were interviewed twice, 6 years apart. Hallstrom and Samuelson (1990) reported on the changes in sexual desire for a subsample of 497 respondents who lived with their partner at the time of both interviews. Present level of sexual desire was assessed using a single item: Respondents characterized their desire as absent, weak, moderate, or strong. Nearly two-thirds of the respondents indicated the same level of sexual interest at both interviews, and very few women indicated an absence of sexual desire. After the age of 50, no respondents reported strong sexual interest, and increasing proportions of women reported little or no sexual desire. By the age of 60, 39% reported no sexual desire. Over the 6-year period, a change of sexual desire was reported by 37% of the women, 27% reported a reduction in sexual interest, and 10% reported an increase. The data indicate some regression to the mean for respondents who had indicated either strong or absent sexual desire at Phase 1 of the study. Respondents who reported strong sexual interest in the first interview later indicated a decline in interest; at the same time, one-half of those who indicated a lack of interest at Phase 1 had regained a weak to moderate sexual desire. A small number of women who indicated a strong, moderate, or weak sexual desire at Phase 1 reported an absence of sexual desire at Phase 2. The results of this study again suggest that for these cohorts of married women, middle-age is characterized by stability of sexual interest rather than by decline, although there was a trend toward decreasing sexual desire for the older cohorts. The declines that were observed were associated with relationship or mental health issues. Similar findings of stability of sexual desire were reported for a comprehensive longitudinal study of sexual behavior in healthy older men and women by the Center for the Study of Aging and Human Development at Duke University (George & Weiler, 1981). Inconsistencies in the literature may be the result of sample differences, including cultural and sociohistorical context, age or health effects, and socioeconomic status, or may result from differences in how researchers define or measure sexual desire and response.

In the recently published text, Kliger and Nedelman (2005) reported on their multiple approaches to research on women's sexual desire and self-esteem. They collected survey data from 408 women in the 50 to 95 age range across the United States, facilitated 10 focus groups with 100+ middle aged and senior women, and conducted in depth interviews with 55 women in this age group. They were interested in how older women age sexually, how women define and perceive sexual desire, and their experiences of sexual desire. Kliger and Nedelman (2006) found that desire tends to diminish with age; more than one-half of their sample experienced a drop in desire, but 40% said that their desire was the same as ever or was even greater. A very small number of respondents did not know what their current level of desire was. The results of this research, although they indicated a loss of desire for many women, may also be interpreted as favoring stability in level of sexual desire.

In an exhaustive review of research on this topic Myers (1995) reported that, although hormones do appear to be important for some aspects of postmenopausal sexuality, hormonal factors only account for a small portion of the variance in the published studies. Myers argued that, based on her meta-analysis, the research from 1972 to 1992 does not support the thesis that women's hormones explain much of the variance in women's sexual response at midlife. Myers commented on the lack of methodological quality in the literature, including the inadequacy of measures, failure to include control groups, and confounding of variables, and she encouraged researchers to expand their definitions of sexuality, to be more complete in their descriptions of methods and results, and to be more attentive to context.

A Critical Perspective on Research on Women's Lack of Desire

Measuring Desire

How do we conceptualize, define, and measure sexual desire in women? Myers (1995) commented on the inadequacy of our measures, and called for more standardization to allow comparisons between samples. In some studies, a single item was used to assess sexual desire; this is clearly inadequate. It is also problematic to use sexual activity as an indicator of desire because, as Kinsey et al. (1953) suggested, coital frequency may reflect men's loss of desire rather than women's. Alternatively, low or decreased coital frequency may be the result of postmenopausal women not having a partner or having a woman partner. Thus, there may not be very close correspondence between women's experience of desire and the frequency of particular forms of sexual activity or women's levels of satisfaction. Furthermore, women may initiate or respond to sexual activity from a state of sexual neutrality (Basson, 2002).

In some studies the measures of sexual desire might reflect an androcentric bias. For example, sexual desire is sometimes operationalized as the number of fantasies or sexual thoughts an individual reports. However, research indicates that women's fantasies are less frequent than men's (Ellis & Symons, 1990). In a community sample of women aged 40 or older, more than one-half of the participants reported no fantasies or one or fewer fantasies (Cutler et al., 1987). Tolman (2001) challenged contemporary constructions of sexuality as limited, male-centered models for health and normalcy and argued that women's experience and understanding of sexual desire differs from that of men. Basson (2002) similarly reviewed evidence that women's sexual desire is experienced differently than men's. Schwartz and Rutter (2000) contended that, for men, who usually initiate the cultural sexual script, their own desire is a sexual cue, but, for many women, the partner's sexual desire is the cue for women's own desire. Women learn to experience their partner's desire as erotic (Schwartz & Rutter, 2000). The research on sexual desire and response in midlife women also reflects heterosexual bias. Researchers have neglected the study of midlife lesbians, and often fail to consider autoerotic activities.

Desire is sometimes seen as synonymous with arousal, but this may be more valid for men than for women. In physically healthy men, genital engorgement is assessed accurately by the individual and this sensation is enjoyed. In women, however, accurate awareness of genital engorgement is lacking. Recent research has indicated that women generally do not separate "desire" from "arousal," and women care more about subjective arousal than they do about physiological arousal. Jill Wood, who studies the sexual responses of women at midlife, found that, although women could distinguish between desire (an interest in sexual activity) and arousal (physical and emotional changes that indicate a readiness for sex), they often used these terms interchangeably. She concluded that women do not conceptualize desire in the same way that researchers have and that women do not distinguish between arousal and desire unless specifically asked to do so (Wood, personal communication, September 30, 2004).

The pharmaceutical industry has recently reported similar findings. Referring to the failure of Viagra to impact women the same way as it impacts men, the *New York Times* (Harris, 2004) reported that Pfizer had recently found that men and women have a fundamentally different relationship between arousal and desire. Women's sexuality was found to be more cognitively complex and less genitally focused than men's. Although Pfizer's researchers viewed this as a disconnect in women between genital changes and mental changes (Harris, 2004), one might also say that the fact that the production of physiological changes in the genitals is enough to impact men's sexual response suggests a simple mechanical response in men.

Tolman (2001) wrote that desire is part of women's embodied and relational self, and she argued for its importance in the understanding of women's sexuality. Desire connects us to our bodies and, at the same time, connects us to another (Tolman, 2001). Yet, women's desire may not be acknowledged, and it is often seen as dangerous in an androcentric culture that emphasizes men's desire and women's responsiveness. These issues can be seen as contributors to women's inability or reluctance to admit to their own sexual desire: "When one is treated as the object of the desires of others, and treats oneself as such, the ability even to know one's own needs and desires is undercut" (Tolman, 2001, p. 199).

Koch (1995, 1997) argued that sexual responding is a complex physiological, psychological, and sociological process. Many social, cultural, religious, and economic factors can affect sexual desire in women. Women may have different and multiple motives for being sexual rather than simply the biologically based desire that many models of sexuality theorize. Women have reported being sexual to enhance emotional closeness and commitment, to express attraction and attractiveness, and to share physical pleasure (Basson, 2002). Women's experience of low levels of desire might result from intimacy problems, the nature of sexual stimuli and stimulation, environmental triggers, and psychological factors that allow or do not allow arousal. A sexual response cycle that incorporates these factors was suggested as an alternative by Basson (2001, 2002), who identified a number of affective, cognitive, and genital feedback loops in women that can contribute to or interfere with sexual "arousability."

What Is Dysfunctional?

The biomedical approach is based on the disease concept, and it labels dissatisfaction and deviation from the norm as dysfunction. Women who do not engage in normative quantities of sexual activity are labeled pathological and dysfunctional (Ogden, 1999; Tiefer, 2001b). The standards established to distinguish between functional and dysfunctional behavior, like definitions of desire, are often based on youthful, heterosexual men's expression as the central criterion of "good" sexual response (Mansfield et al., 1998). Conceptions of function and dysfunction are grounded in biological perspectives of sexuality, which do not consider women's unique sociocultural position with regard to sexual desire and expression (Richgels, 1992). For example, criteria for the diagnosis of hypoactive sexual desire fail to consider the ways in which women's sexuality is repressed and criticized. Further, Richgels argued that the norms for women's sexual response have varied greatly through history, and have generally not corresponded to women's actual experiences. Norms for healthy or satisfying sexuality for older women based on the experiences of older women have not been established. Feminist sexologists (e.g., Irvine, 1990; Tiefer, 1995) have urged researchers to use measures that focus on women's pleasure. Others have suggested that menopause actually represents, for some women, the opportunity to define their sexuality based on their own desires and needs rather than on soicocultural expectations of reproduction and the satisfaction of marital duties (Barbach, 1975; Conway-Turner, 1992; Laws, 1980). Bancroft et al. (2003) have questioned whether we should label older women as dysfunctional when they have less sexual interest than they had when they were younger. They argued that the label of sexual dysfunction should rely heavily on the woman's own construction of her sexuality, rather than on the researchers' standardized criteria for what constitutes functional and dysfunctional sex. Midlife women may be sexually satisfied despite any sexual changes they experience (Avis et al., 1995; Bancroft et al., 2003). Across four studies reviewed by Bancroft et al., only one-third to one-half of the women who were defined as having a problem by the research criteria regarded themselves as having a problem. Lessened sexual response did not concern most of the older women (Koch et al., 1995; Bancroft et al., 2003). As long as couples still are sexually active, and it is not unpleasant, the pairs believe that they are meeting a requirement of marriage (Schwartz & Rutter, 2000). In research conducted by Osborn et al. (1988), English women did report having sexual problems. However, their conceptions of the sexual problems differed from the operational definition of the researchers. For example, lack of emotional well-being and emotional feelings during sexual interaction with a partner were more important determinants of sexual distress from the women's point of view. These discrepancies between the respondents' and the researchers' conceptions of problems emphasizes the question: Who gets to define or determine who has a sexual problem? Who sets the criteria for having enough or too much sexual activity or desire?

Is absence or reduction in sexual desire or sexual activity a dysfunction? The question "When is it appropriate to call a pattern of behavior a sexual problem or a dysfunction?" has been raised repeatedly (Bancroft et al., 2003; McHugh, in press; Tiefer, 2001b). Bancroft et al. (2003) found no significant relationship between age and self-defined "problems." In their research, it was younger women who were more likely to report nonpleasurable sex, sexual anxiety, and pain during sex. The authors suggested that, in at least some cases, inhibition of sexual desire is an adaptive mechanism (Bancroft et al., 2003). This may be because the greater experience and confidence that comes with aging mean that women are more likely to refuse nonpleasurable sex and less likely to be sexually anxious.

According to Koch et al. (2005) midlife women tend to be sexually satisfied regardless of the sexual changes they report. The effects of aging on the levels of sexual interest of women in their study were not a cause of concern. Sexual thoughts were reported less frequently by older women, but that was not necessarily seen as problematic. Older women seemed to have more sexual problems (as defined by the researchers) but less distress over them. The women who were not having partner sex were older and masturbated more frequently; they reported more distress about their relationship or lack thereof, but not about their own sexuality. This finding is consistent with Conway-Turner's conclusion that quality of intimacy, more than frequency of sexual intercourse, is important to African American senior women and positively related to their sexual self-esteem (Conway-Turner, 1992).

Laumann et al. (1999) reported that 43% of American women suffer from a sexual problem, yet the problems encountered were most often associated with mental health, relationship problems, and various aspects of the quality of life than with physiologically based desire and arousal. The women's levels of distress about their relationship and their own sexuality were related both to their physical and mental health. Their own physical health was a direct determinant of women's feelings about their own sexuality; older women with lubrication problems reported marked distress about their own sexuality.

The research reviewed above reiterates the importance of conceptualizing the sexual problems of women differently than those of men. The findings also suggest the importance of the contextual factors. Women's well-being, physical health, level of education, and relationship to their partner predicted whether they were experiencing distress. Factors about the relationship including communication, intimacy, and respect are good predictors of women's sexual satisfaction (Koch et al., 2005). "While it is good to encourage older couples to maintain and foster their sexual intimacy, should we be encouraging older women to regard themselves as dysfunctional because they have less sexual interest than when they were younger?" (Bancroft et al., 2003, p. 502).

Foucault (1978) viewed desire as socially constructed rather than merely perceived; in his theory desires are not biological entities, but are produced within social practices and cultural discourses. From this perspective sexual desire is a cultural product, and it is produced or constructed differently in different societies and historical periods. Richgels (1992) reviewed the history of cultural perspectives on women's sexual desire or lack thereof from the Victorians' denial of women's sexual feelings to contemporary prescriptions of "sex experts." She argued that modern views in which women's lack of desire is seen as dysfunctional are as limiting as the Victorian conception of women's desire as disease. Currently social and medical views privilege heterosexual intercourse and men's sexual desire as normative, rendering women's sexual pleasure, especially in the form of self pleasuring and lesbian partner sexual interactions, invisible, dysfunctional, and devalued (Richgels, 1992).

The Medicalization of Desire

Following the financial success of Viagra, the pharmaceutical industry instigated a search for a new market for their drug: women. Tiefer (2001a) and Moynihan (2001) have revealed the drug industry's attempt to repeat the medicalization process so successful with men's sexuality with regard to women's sexuality. Tiefer alerted us to the construction of the new diagnosis "female sexual dysfunction" (FSD). She exposed this process as a rush to medicalize women's sexual problems in order to turn women's sexual problems into drug company profits. Multiple arguments against such a medicalized view of women's sexuality can be read in *A New View of Women's Sexual Problems*, a volume edited by Kaschak and Tiefer (2001). The contributors contest a medicalized view of sexuality and challenge the reduction of women's sexuality to a series of movements, muscles spasms, or moving parts.

Currently, the industry's search for a cure for women's sexual problems is focused on hypoactive sexual desire, defined as persistent and pervasive inhibition of sexual desire (American Psychiatric Association, 1994). Assessment of hypoactive sexual desire assumes an accepted standard of normal sexual appetite (Richgels, 1992).

Richgels (1992) views the diagnosis of hypoactive sexual desire as a cultural construction that contributes to the control of women's sexuality. She argued that this diagnostic label fails to view women's sexuality in the context of contemporary American culture in which men's sexuality is privileged. According to Richgels, medical and psychological labels fail to consider women's experience of sexuality not only as pleasure, but also as possible danger (Vance, 1984).

In an attempt to find a pharmaceutical solution to the diagnosed problem of hypoactive sexual desire, testosterone, the hormone that allegedly fuels men's sexual appetite, is being investigated for its ability to increase sexual desire in (postmenopausal) women. Procter and Gamble began a public relations campaign touting the benefits of the experimental testosterone patch. In the *British Medical Journal*, Moynihan (2004) revealed that Procter and Gamble had designed, funded, and even conducted themselves the research that "documented" the effectiveness of the patch in increasing the sexual responsiveness of surgically menopausal women. The research was reported in the mainstream press, but was not submitted to the standard peer review required for scientific publication. Moynihan's critique regarding the press reports of the effects of the patch include: exaggerating the benefits of the patch; inflating the pool of potential candidates (to all women with low sexual desire); minimizing the potential for harm from hormone use; ignoring the issue of conflict of interest when the supporting research is supplied by the producer of the product. To date, no pharmaceutical treatment for women's sexual response "problem" has been approved by the U.S. Food and Drug Administration.

The adoption of a pharmaceutical/medical approach to women's experiences has limited, distorted, and pathologized women's sexuality. Tiefer and her colleagues (Kaschak & Tiefer, 2001; Tiefer, 2001a) have exposed the medicalization of sexuality as an active process, even a strategy, devised by groups with political and socioeconomic interests best served by the medical model. *The New View Campaign* (Kaschak & Tiefer, 2001; Working Group on Women's Sexual Problems, n.d.) has enumerated several problems with the medicalization of sexual desire. The medicalization of a condition is to make it a disease, the cure for which, a pharmaceutical prescription, becomes the first line of defense. The seemingly neutral and scientific language of "disease" can offer a palpable relief to those who secretly worry that their sexuality is inadequate. People respond to the diagnosis of a disease with relief because the diagnosis of the problem suggests that it is located within the individual's biochemistry. The individual (patient) then relies on the efficacy of the medicine rather than relying on life circumstances or lifestyle changes, which might have either prevented or alleviated the condition in the first place.

The medical model erases the relational context of sexuality. The medical emphasis on sexual physiology and performance reinforces narrow definitions of sexuality, and it diminishes styles of sexuality that do not focus on genital arousal and orgasm. The medical model and its practitioners ignore women's complex sexualities, and give women more reasons to feel insecure. Further, subscription to the medical perspective is likely to result in less emphasis on sex education efforts, and may cause insurance companies to endorse pharmaceutical solutions and to limit reimbursement for counseling (Tiefer, 2001b). The emphasis on physiological functions and pharmaceutical solutions may contribute to the media, medical practitioners, and patients ignoring social and cultural factors. Under the medical model, factors that are more likely to be sources of women's sexual complaints (e.g., relational issues, sexual ignorance, or fear) are downplayed and dismissed (McHugh, in press).

A medical perspective on women's sexuality may fail to address differences among women, as it generally ignores the implications of inequalities created by gender, race, class, and sexual orientation (Working Group on Women's Sexual Problems). The medical model ignores diversity, reducing all women to a single set of physiological responses, symptoms, dysfunctions, and causes. In contrast, feminist approaches within sociology, sexology, and psychology recognize that women are not a homogenous group and that women's sexuality is not a single or simplistic phenomenon. Conceptions of desire, attraction, arousal, and satisfaction are complex constructions that develop in a sociohistorical context, and are impacted by race/ethnicity, age, religious orientation, geographic region, socioeconomic class, age cohort, and even neighborhood (McHugh, in press; Tiefer, 1995) A medical model that views genital and physiological processes as identical across women (and as basically the same for men and for women) ignores the implications of inequalities related to gender, social class, ethnicity, and sexual orientation. Women over 50 are a diverse group whose sexuality and intimate relations are multifaceted and dynamic.

The Context of Women's Sexuality

Women of the 1950s

The research reviewed above documented that declines in sexual activity and desire may not be easily applied to the current generation of women in their 50s. The research on women's sexuality at menopause reported in the 1980s describe data based on women born in 1935 or earlier, who came of age in the 1950s. Those respondents, if still living, would be in their 70s or 80s today. As previously mentioned, the literature that stresses physiology as the basis for women's sexual desire emphasizes universals and fails to consider the sociohistorical or cultural context of women's experience.

Women's sexual experiences can best be understood in the cultural context of their lives. Women in their early 50s today were born in the 1950s. Although they were born in a socially conservative era, they came of age in the late 1960s and early 1970s, a time of alleged sexual liberation. Born in 1952, I am from this generation, the generation of so-called "free love." My generation had access to the birth control pill in our late teens and to legal abortion for most of our reproductive lives. Some of us took Women's Studies or assertiveness classes, attended consciousness-raising groups, and participated in the women's health movement. Some of us held mirrors to our genitals to learn about our bodies, and many of us owned copies of the original *Our Bodies Ourselves* (Boston Women's Health Book Collective, 1976). Women in their 50s today have generally benefited from the Women's Health Movement. We lived through multiple epidemics of sexually transmitted diseases, and were adults when awareness of AIDS surfaced. Our experiences of intimacy and desire, and our constructions of our sexuality as middle-aged women is probably different from those of our mothers at age 50. My mother, for example, was born in 1924, came of age during World War II, and turned 50 in 1974. Even after having returned to school in her 50s and having earned a college degree and a Women's Studies certificate, she chooses not to speak about sex.

A woman's sense of herself as a sexual being, her thoughts about the meaning of sex, and her awareness of her own sexual desire are all constructed in a particular sociohistorical context. Each generation has to define itself sexually, and young people continually rewrite the sexual stories told by their elders (Trafford, 1995). Sexual practices and the terms used to label them are dynamic rather than static. Sexual experiences and practices are impacted by changing times, and yet is there is also continuity to the human experience. Although she acknowledged that in the second half of the twentieth century Western societies have experienced the consequences of wide spread contraceptive practices, the economic emancipation of women, feminism, and sexual liberation on an unprecedented scale, Fonatana

(1994) critiqued the belief that the problems we are confronting today are radically new ones, unknown in previous generations. There are both continuities and differences in the experiences of generations.

Even within a specific historical era women's experiences are diverse. Women's sexuality is impacted by a number of factors, including geographic region, class, ethnicity, sexual orientation, and history of violence. Older women, like younger women, vary enormously in their sexual desire, arousal, and experience of orgasm (Leiblum, 1990). The context of her life also influences what a woman knows/thinks about menopause and aging.

Relationship Context

Research has demonstrated that marital status is an important predictor of decreased sexual activity (Mansfield et al., 1995). Kinsey et al. (1953) attributed the decrease in coital frequency of a couple to the male partner's declining interest in sociosexual activities. Because older women often have even older partners, it is not safe to assume that decreased sexual activity is related to women's desire, much less related to women's hormone levels. Thus, Bachman (1990) concluded that the sexual activity of a heterosexual woman is dictated by the availability, functioning, and desire of her male partner.

In the Midlife Survey (Mansfield et al.), marital status, not menopausal status predicted desire and enjoyment; the longer the marital relationship, the less desire and enjoyment was reported. Furthermore, being married rather than single was associated with a decline of sexual responsiveness, but menopausal status was not. In other research, women's sexual activity also was strongly related to marital status (Diokno et al., 1990), and women indicated that their husbands were the reason they were no longer engaging in sexual activities (Pfeiffer et al., 1972). Decreases in sexual desire were associated with a poor relationship with one's spouse, with life stress events, and with mental disorder, major depression, and use of psychotropic medicine (Hallstrom & Samuelson, 1990). Similarly, Bancroft et al. (2003) reported that, in their large study of heterosexual women aged 20 to 64, age had only a modest effect in predicting sexual distress regarding the relationship or one's own sexuality. Lack of emotional well-being and emotional feelings during sexual interaction with the partner were more important determinants of sexual distress. In a number of well-designed studies factors associated with the quality of life and aspects of the relationship have been shown to predict sexual satisfaction for women (Koch et al., 2005).

Other researchers have reported a strong positive correlation between sexual satisfaction and relationship satisfaction for the middle-aged and older women in their samples; sexual satisfaction has also been positively correlated with passionate love (Traupmann et al., 1982). This research suggests that when relationship satisfaction is low, so is sexual satisfaction. As previously cited, Mansfield et al. (1995, 1998) concluded that marriage, rather than menopausal status, was associated with sexual response declines. Youthful men's sexual experience may continue to serve as the sexual norm that both women and men use to judge the quality of their sexual response.

For many women desire is experienced in the context of a relationship. Their own desire is experienced in relation to their attractiveness to a partner. Thus, their desire mirrors their partner's desire. Schwartz and Rutter (2000) suggested that women are trained to value commitment, and they may rely less on erotic stimulation, and more on relationship satisfaction, as the basis for sexual arousal. Some widows have said when their spouse died, their desire faded; yet other women have found desire in a new relationship. Older women's descriptions of their needs and desires in a qualitative study by Wood et al. (in press) suggested that some women had internalized a cultural ideology that privileged their male partner's needs over their own. Some women were disappointed with their partner's technique and had experienced sex as unsatisfying and work-like, but the women felt an obligation to attend to their partner's needs. Other women reported that they avoided sex to protect their partner from the embarrassment of erectile dysfunction. The women generally did not have the ability to express their own sexual desires and needs. The quality of the women's relationship with their husbands was the most frequently cited influence on their own experience of sexual desire.

Marital relationships, as well as the individuals in them, go through developmental changes over time. Relationships need to grow and develop as do the individuals involved. There may be an ebb and flow to marital sexual relations that is not considered in culturally prescriptive norms. According to Schwartz and Rutter (2000), declining sexual activity among older adults may be more related to the length of the relationship and habituation than to aging. "Couples evolve into partners rather than lovers" (Schwartz & Rutter, 2000, p. 132). The sex lives of 50- and 60-year-old newlyweds resemble the sex lives of younger couples more than they do the sex lives of long-married couples of the same age, and their active sex lives follow the same pattern of eventual decline (Blumstein & Schwartz, 1983). In most marriages, sex becomes less frequent, but not less pleasant, over time (Schwartz & Rutter, 2000).

Relationship conflicts have been noted as a common source of sexual problems (Leiblum, 1990). Women have reported various relationship problems, including a lack of spontaneity, initiative, or romance. Complaints about the personal hygiene and appearance of the partner are not uncommon (Leiblum, 1990), and couples with well established sexual routines may find that they no longer elicit much excitement or interest. Butler and Lewis (1976) reported that relationship issues, including boredom, too much togetherness, illness, or problems with hygiene, may be expressed as pain during intercourse, perhaps because pain is a more acceptable "excuse" for limiting sexual activities.

In their study of women's sexual response at midlife, Mansfield et al. (1998) found that the 40% of women who reported changes in their sexual response reported less sexual interest. Women indicated that they wanted more fulfilling sexual relationships. The women wanted to become more passionate, more interested in sex, more romantic, more affectionate, more communicative, more sexually responsive, more desirous of sex, more initiating, more fun, more creative, less boring, more loving, and less inhibited. They wanted their husbands to be more communicative, more romantic, more affectionate, more fun, more passionate, more loving, more creative, and less boring. The biomedical approach, with its focus on changes in physiological responsiveness, has ignored women's stated desire for more communication and affection in their relationships.

Women's sexual functioning has been shown to be impacted by partner factors, such as presence of a partner, feelings toward the partner, and partner's health (Dennerstein et al., 2001). The research by Dennerstein et al. (1999, 2001) confirmed the effects of aging and menopause, yet the authors stressed that women's relationships with their partners had particularly powerful effects on women's sexual desire. In research by Ellison and Zilbergeld (as cited in Ellison, 2001) the top three items associated with satisfying sex for women were: feeling close to a partner before sex, emotional closeness after sexual activity, and feeling loved. Similarly, Byers (2001) presented empirical research that indicates that relationship satisfaction is the most important contributor to women's sexual satisfaction, more important than the types of sexual exchanges such as oral sex, the consistency of orgasm, and the expression of affection, which are all important determinants of women's sexual satisfaction. An earlier study of 100 married couples (Frank et al., 1978) showed that, although 80% of the couples labeled their marriages and sexual relationships as satisfying, 43% of the men and 63% of the women reported arousal or orgasmic difficulties. High levels of additional concerns were also indicated, such as lack of interest or inability to relax (Frank et al., 1978). These and other descriptions of women's sexuality confirm the perspective that women's sexual satisfaction is connected to the relationship context. Ellison stated that her survey results support the following conclusion: that women associate sexual satisfaction in relationships with closeness, love, acceptance, and safety, and that the sexual problems and concerns of women often center on intimacy and relationship issues.

Partners Using Viagra

A few researchers who recognized the importance of relationships to women's experience of sexual desire and satisfaction have examined the impact of Viagra use by male partners on heterosexual women's sexual experiences. Potts et al. (2003) drew on interviews with 27 women, age 33 and 68, in a New Zealand study to identify issues and concern for women regarding their partners' use of Viagra. Most women reported that use of Viagra had altered some aspects of their sexual relationship, including increased frequency of intercourse, prolonged duration of sexual relations, and less experience of nonpenetrative aspects of intimacy. These effects were not always desired by women; even women who had a generally positive reaction saw the increased frequency of coitus as a drawback. Some women reported discomfort, pain, and cystitis. Similarly, Riley and Riley (2000) found that one-half of women partners of Viagra users expressed a preference for activities other than penile–vaginal sex. Like the women interviewed by Wood et al.

(in press), the New Zealand women reported "putting up" with sex and engaging in coital sex when they did not desire it. Both sets of authors commented on the problems women had negotiating with their partners concerning when to have sex and in which type of sexual and intimate activities to engage. Although some women have had difficulty negotiating with their partners regarding the use of Viagra, other women have used Viagra as the occasion to speak out about women's sexuality and to offer critical comments on the medical industry (Loe, 2004).

Lesbian Couples

The heterosexual bias in existing research on older women's sexual functioning has often been criticized. The research that suggests that length of relationship predicts the frequency of sexual relations and that satisfaction with the relationship predicts sexual satisfaction is all based on heterosexual couples. In a unique study of menopausal lesbians, Cole and Rothblum (1991) concluded that lesbians are more positive about sex than their heterosexual counterparts are. The sample of 41 sexually active lesbians willing to talk about sex may not represent the population of menopausal lesbians, but the results suggest that sexual orientation is an important consideration in women's sexuality at midlife. For example, the respondents in the Cole and Rothblum's study did not report declines in sexual satisfaction and activity.

Winterich (2003) used a qualitative approach to examine the social aspects of women's sexuality after menopause in a sample that included both heterosexual and lesbian women. She found that, in some cases, both lesbian and heterosexual women had active and fulfilling sex lives. For her participants, although changes in desire or orgasm or vaginal dryness might have occurred, their sexual relations and satisfaction were not negatively affected. Open communication with their partners and a flexibility regarding sexual repertoire was present in the sexually satisfied couples, regardless of orientation. Among the women who reported sexual problems, heterosexual women described issues that were related to the cultural constructions of menopause, gender roles, and heterosexual sex. For example, some of the heterosexual women reported faked orgasms, partners' complaints about their vaginal dryness, and an inability to talk to their partners about what they wanted. Although some of the lesbians did report sexual problems, they also reported the ability to discuss their needs and issues with their partners. Several lesbian and heterosexual women were not having sex for a variety of reasons, including not being in a relationship, healing from past trauma, and current relationship problems.

In addition to including nonheterosexual options for sexual pleasure, Winterich's (2003) research emphasizes the need to consider how women view menopause rather than just to focus on menopause as a problem, or as the cause of sexual dissatisfaction. In women's own accounts of sex after menopause, the status and quality of relationships and their own and their partner's health were important factors for both lesbian and heterosexual women.

Cultural Attitudes Toward Women's Bodies and Attractiveness

In our society, older women and their bodies are frequently denigrated or rendered invisible, and it is the norm for women to be dissatisfied with their bodies (Banister, 1999; Koch et al., 2005). We often fail to see older women as sexy and sexual. Others have critiqued the double standard of aging, that is, the cultural belief that women become less attractive and less sexually appealing as they age, whereas men do not (Bernard, 1981). Women's sense of themselves as attractive has been demonstrated to impact their perceptions of sexuality. Frequency of sexual behaviors is related to ratings of attractiveness and body satisfaction in some research (Faith & Schare, 1993). Anderson and LeGrand (1991) found that women with unfavorable evaluations of their bodies engaged in a more restricted range of sexual activities than did those with a favorable attitude. Women with poor body images reported more problems with sexual desire. Fooken (1994) found that, for the West German women in her sample, a positive body image helped to maintain satisfactory levels of sexual desire. In the research conducted by Klinger and Nedelman (2005) over 50% of women listed negative changes in their body image as the primary factor in decreased sexual desire. The authors reported that women who continue to feel positive about themselves as sexual beings adjusted well to their altered bodies.

Women's body image has an impact on their sexual desire, experience of orgasm, sexual enjoyment, and frequency of sexual relations, but not on their sexual satisfaction. Koch et al. (2005) reported that the more a woman perceived herself as less attractive now than 10 years ago, the more likely she was to report a decline in sexual desire or frequency of sexual activity. The more attractive she perceived herself to be, the more likely she was to experience an increase in sexual desire, orgasm, sexual enjoyment, or frequency of sexual activity.

According to Taylor and Sumrall (1993), many of the accounts they collected from 66 spirited women over 40 concerning women's sexuality at midlife and beyond shatter the stereotypes that the public and the media hold about older women and their bodies. Although women often experienced wrinkles, weight gain, and other bodily changes, most of them did not spend their time and money trying to recapture their youth. Research indicates that, although body dissatisfaction remained stable across the age range of 20 to 84, related behaviors, such as body monitoring, appearance anxiety, and self-objectification, declined with age (Tiggerman & Lynch, 2002). For some women, maturation includes movement away from concerns about culturally valued beauty, femininity, and sex appeal.

Giesen (1989) explored 32 women's perceptions of their own attractiveness, femininity, and sex appeal, currently and in relation to 10 years ago. The respondents ranged in age from 28 to 63 and were both married and single. The findings indicate that attractiveness was defined by physical attributes, femininity by behaviors and traits, and sex appeal was defined equally by physical features and behaviors. Marriage mediated the degree to which older women viewed themselves as attractive and sexually appealing.

Single women, but not married women, viewed themselves as having grown more attractive, feminine, and sexually appealing as they aged. Single women saw themselves as having grown more attractive and more sexually appealing over the past 10 years, and they saw the peak years of women's attractiveness as occurring in the early 30s to early 50s. Older married women saw women's peak attractiveness as occurring in their early 20s.

Other Contextual Factors

Recent feminist analyses of women's sexual problems have emphasized the lack of sexual information, cultural attitudes and messages, family and work stress, partner and relationship issues, and psychological factors such as depression and anxiety (Kaschak & Tiefer, 2001; McHugh, in press). Life stressors and other contextual factors including cultural prescriptions regarding sexual activity in later life are likely to impact women's sexual functioning at midlife (Mansfield et al., 1995). The women in the research conducted by Wood et al. (in press) reported that stress from various parts of their lives was an important determinant of sexual desire. Dennerstein et al. (2001) reported that social factors, including educational level, experience of stress, and daily hassles, affected sexual functioning. Laumann et al. (1999) emphasized the impact of mental health and quality of life on the experience of sexual problems. The three most often reported (negative) sexual experiences of the respondents in the Ellison and Zilbergeld study were being too tired to have sex, being too busy, and having lower sexual desire than they wanted to have (Ellison, 2001). Candib (2001) similarly reported that her clients, who are low-income, multiethnic women, often express a lack of interest in sex, and report "not feeling anything." She suggested that the cause of their problems is not biology, but the lived experience of working two jobs, doing child care, and managing a household. Working women are often too tired to be interested in sex, according to Candib (2001). Thus, the ultimate solution to women's sexual problems may be more time, less stress, better education, and more attentive partners (Shah, 2001).

Variability and Possibility

Gynocentric Research

Androcentrism, the valuing or privileging of men's experience, has repeatedly been acknowledged as problematic in the conceptualization of women's sexual desire and response. In her discussion of the heterosexual bias in our constructions of women's sexuality Marrow (1997) labeled the maps of the sexual journey provided by popular culture as "faulty, showing a freeway to heterosexual marriage, penile–vaginal intercourse, childbearing and a loss of sexuality in old age" (p. xi). Others too have commented on the cultural emphasis on being pleasing and accessible to men. Daniluk (1998) presented exercises and other techniques for "helping women to extricate themselves from the oppressive shoulds and should nots . . . of our dominant sexual scripts" (p. 231). She argued that our culture does not have ways of constructing sexual expression that "affirm women's sexual agency and the diversity of their sexual feelings and desire" (p. 221).

Researchers' conceptions of sexual desire and response may or may not correspond with or include women's own construction of their sexual desire and response. For example, the responses that women gave to open-ended questions about sexuality caused some researchers to begin to include questions about nongenital as well as genital sexual expression (Mansfield et al., 2000). Research that uses interviews, narratives, or other approaches to study women's experience of sexuality from their own points of view does not produce accounts that correspond to Masters and Johnson's sexual response cycle (Masters & Johnson, 1966). The response cycle of Masters and Johnson does not address the relationship context of sexual experiences; yet women's experience of sexuality is more relationship-oriented and less genitally focused that men's (Conway-Turner, 1992; Peplau & Gordon, 1985). Women appear to desire greater intimacy than men do (Tiefer, 1995), and they value physical affection and nongenital intimacy more than men do (Blumstein & Schwartz, 1983; Mansfield et al., 1998). Consistent with this perspective, the New View campaign has called for research and services "driven not by commercial interests, but by women's own needs and sexual realities" (Working Group on Women's Sexual Problems, n.d.).

Hetero-normative Prescriptions

The universalizing and homogenizing aspects of the biomedical approach may have detrimental effects on women and on the sexuality research agenda. Although women want to be informed about what to expect, the presentation of certain outcomes as likely can become prescriptive or self-fulfilling. As Irvine (1990) pointed out, sex is a social product; it is negotiated and constructed through discursive practices, including educational texts as well as advertising and self-help manuals. Sexuality is organized through regulation and definition. The conception that hormones are responsible for a decline in sexual desire and activity may relieve some women, but can become an expectation in others that is negative and self-fulfilling. On the other hand, in attempting to overcome the cultural belief that older women are not sexual, psychologists' and others' encouragement to remain or become passionate (Sheehy, 2006) may be experienced as pressure to engage in unwanted sexual activities. To document and publicize norms regarding older women's sexual response is sometimes to provide a cultural prescription. Women may be criticized when their sexual desire exceeds cultural expectations (Ogden, 1999), and they may be labeled dysfunctional when their interest in sex falls below the (androcentric and youthful) norms. It can feel like a no-win situation.

Sexual Authenticity

Miller (1976) argued that sexual authenticity is a key feature of women's psychological health. She identified sexual authenticity as the ability to bring one's own real feelings of sexual desire and sexual pleasure into intimate relationships. Authenticity distinguishes women who feel disoriented in their aging bodies from women who are confident and sexually secure. Alternatively, Tolman (2002) refers to a similar concept, sexual subjectivity, which is to experience oneself as a sexual being, to be in touch with one's own sexual desire. Several authors (e.g., Martin, 1996; Richgels, 1992; Tolman, 2002)) have noted that it is a challenge in an androcentric society for women to exercise sexual agency, that is, the ability to recognize and act on one's own desire and to experience sexual pleasure. Women's ability to recognize their own sexual desire and to negotiate on their own behalf was also emphasized in recent approaches (e.g., Wood et al., in press; Potts et al., 2003; Kliger & Nedelman, 2006). Women's ability to act on their own behalf (also called negotiated sexual agency) was identified as a core variable in women's experience of sexual desire in qualitative research conducted with postmenopausal women (Wood et al., in press). Thus, the application of homogenized prescriptions and androcentric standards to women's sexual desire and response works against the goal of helping women to be in touch with themselves and to be comfortable with their own levels of desire and activity. Researchers may contribute to women's experience of sexual authenticity at midlife by examining women's own conceptions and experiences of desire and by emphasizing the variability and potential of women's sexual experiences rather than assuming a physiologically based, homogenized, and declining sexual desire.

Variability

Kinsey et al. (1953) emphasized the variability in the human sexual response and noted that diversity is the single most identifiable aspect of sexuality. Leiblum (1990) observed that women, at all ages, vary enormously in sexual desire, sexual satisfaction, orgasmic experience, and arousability. Similarly, Kliger and Nedelman (2005) argued that there is not a single best or right way for women at any age to express their sexuality. The women they surveyed reported multiple and diverse sexual responses. Many older women have a fulfilling, exciting, and creative life without any sexual desire or sexual activity, whereas others report increased appreciation for sensual experiences as they age. In each of the studies reviewed above there was at least a small percentage of women for whom desire increased in the senior years, and, for others, desire remained as a steady state. Kliger and Nedelman (2006) concluded that sexual desire waxes and wanes over time. The changes women experience in sexual desire and activity may relate to other aspects of their lives or may have no clear trigger or influence (e.g., stress levels, ages of children).

At age 50, as at all other ages, women may express their sexuality in varied ways. Variability is experienced by both married and single, heterosexual and lesbian women (Kliger & Nedelman, 2006). A similar conclusion can be reached by reading the personal accounts collected by Taylor and Sumrall (1993). They present stories, personal accounts, and poems written by women over 40 about women's sexuality at midlife and beyond. Their text attests to the diversity of women's experiences. The new edition of *Our Bodies, Ourselves* (Boston Women's Health Book Collective, 2005) also enumerates some of the experiences of women as they age including increased sexual desire, changes in sexual preference, feeling removed from sexual practices and urges, finding alternatives to traditional relationships, appreciating a non sexual sensuality, and recognizing an awakening of old feelings. Ellison (2001) similarly concluded that women can experience sexual pleasure in a variety of ways. Each woman has the capacity to respond sexually in a variety of ways, and she is likely to experiences changes during her lifetime in how she experiences her body, her relationships, and her sexual desire. Women's sexuality at all ages is multifaceted, complex, and dynamic. To evaluate the adequacy of women's sexuality against a single standard or on a single dimension seems senseless.

Several recent texts concern the variability and the dynamic nature of women's sexuality over the lifespan and encourage women to respect their own experience, rather than to subscribe to normative and pharmaceutical prescriptions. Kliger and Nedelman (2006) and Sheehy (2006) emphasized women's passion and diverse sexual options after 50, explicitly countering the homogenized view of older women as lacking in desire and desirability. Some women at midlife are more self-actualized and more willing to explore, and perhaps redefine, what feels right sexually rather than conforming to a coitally focused model of sexuality (Mansfield et al., 2000; Tiefer, 1995). Cole (1988) encouraged therapists to provide women with permission to have different, more mature kinds of sex lives and to help women to develop an expanded view of sexuality and sensuality. The Boston Women's Health Book Collective (2005) encouraged women to recognize that lovemaking may become more enjoyable when they no longer are concerned with pregnancy and have more privacy at home. Some women enjoy lovemaking more as a result of years of a committed relationship. Some women, such as Betty Dodson, have relationships with younger men. Others have sexual relationships with women for the first time.

Viewing women's sexuality from androcentric, heterosexist, and biomedical perspectives has limited the types of research questions we have asked, and has impacted the methodologies employed in the conduct of research. Challenges to existing research paradigms have suggested new research questions and strategies. Future research on the sexual experiences and feelings of women at midlife might entertain multiple perspectives and allow for positive changes as well as declines or loss of function. Increasingly theorists are recognizing the need to conduct gynocentric research on women's experience and to recognize the variability among women. Researchers, like the women they are studying, might increasingly examine the sexual possibilities that arise from developmental transitions in women's lives.

References

American Psychiatric Association. (1994). *Diagnostic and Statistical Manual of Mental Disorders* (4th ed.). Washington, DC: Author.

Anderson, B.L., and LeGrand, J. (1991). Body image for women: Conceptualization, assessment, and a test of its importance to sexual dysfunction and medical illness. *Journal of Sex Research, 28*, 457–477.

Avis, N.E., Stellato, R., Crawford, S., and Johannes, C. (1995). How does menopause impact sexual activity? *Menopause, 2*, 245.

Bachmann, G., Leiblum, S., and Grill, J. (1989). Brief sexual inquiry in gynecologic practice. *Obstetrics & Gynecology, 73*, 425–427.

Bancroft, J., Loftus, J., and Long, J.S. (2003). Distress about sex: A national survey of women in heterosexual relationships. *Archives of Sexual Behavior, 32*, 193–209.

Banister, E.M. (1999). Women's midlife experience of their changing bodies. *Qualitative Health Research, 9*, 520–537.

Barbach, L. (1975). *For Yourself: The Fulfillment of Female Sexuality*. New York: Anchor Books.

Basson, R. (2001). Human sex response cycles. *Journal of Sex and Marital Therapy, 27*, 33–43.

Basson, R. (2002). Women's sexual desire: Disordered or misunderstood. *Journal of Sex and Marital Therapy, 28*(Suppl), 17–28.

Bernard, J. (1981). *The Female World*. New York: Free Press.

Blumstein, P., and Schwartz, P. (1983). *American Couples*. New York: Morrow.

Boston Women's Health Book Collective. (1976). *Our Bodies, Ourselves*. Boston: Touchstone.

Boston Women's Health Book Collective. (2005). *Our Bodies, Ourselves*. Boston: Touchstone.

Butler, R.N., and Lewis, M.I. (1976). *Sex After Sixty*. New York: Harper & Row.

Byers, E.S. (2001). Evidence for the importance of relationship satisfaction for women's sexual functioning. In E. Kaschak and L. Tiefer (Eds.), *A New View of Women's Sexual Problems* (pp. 23–26). Binghamton, NY: Haworth Press.

Candib, L.M. (2001). "A new view of women's sexual problems": A family physician's response. In E. Kaschak and L. Tiefer (Eds.), *A New View of Women's Sexual Problems* (pp. 9–15). Binghamton, NY: Haworth Press.

Cole, E. (1988). Sex at menopause: Each in her own way. *Women & Therapy, 7*(2/3), 159–168.

Cole, E. and Rothblum, E.D. (1991). Lesbian sex at menopause: As good as or better than ever. In B. Sang, J. Warshaw, and A. Smith (Eds.), *Lesbians at Midlife: The Creative Transition* (pp. 184–193). San Francisco, CA: Spinsters Ink.

Conway-Turner, K. (1992). Sex, intimacy, and self-esteem: The case of the African American older woman. *Women & Aging, 4*, 91–104.

Cutler, W.B., Garcia, C.R., and McCoy, N. (1987). Perimenopausal sexuality. *Archives of Sexual Behavior, 16*, 225–234.

Daniluk, J.C. (1998). *Women's Sexuality Across the Lifespan: Challenging Myths, Creating Meanings*. New York: Guilford.

Dennerstein, L., Alexander, J.L., and Kotz, K. (2003). The menopause and sexual functioning: A review of the population-based studies. *Annual Review of Sex Research, 14*, 64–82.

Dennerstein, L., Dudley, E., and Burger, H. (2001). Are changes in sexual functioning during midlife due to aging or menopause? *Fertility & Sterility, 76*, 456–460.

Dennerstein, L. Dudley, E. Hopper, J., and Burger, H. (1997). Sexuality, hormones and the menopausal transition. *Maturitas, 26*, 83–93.

Dennerstein, L., Lehert, P., Burger, H., and Dudley, E. (1999). Factors affecting sexual functioning of women in the midlife years. *Climateric, 2*, 254–262.

Diokno, A.C., Brown, M.B., and Rugula-Herzog, A. (1990). Sexual function in the elderly. *Archives of Internal Medicine, 150*, 197–200.

Ellis, B.J., and Symons, D. (1990). Sex differences in sexual fantasy: An evolutionary psychological approach. *Journal of Sex Research, 27*, 527–555.

Ellison, C.R. (2001). A research inquiry into some American women's sexual concerns and problems. In E. Kaschak and L. Tiefer (Eds.), *A New View of Women's Sexual Problems* (pp. 147–160). Binghamton, NY: Haworth Press.

Faith, M.S., and Schare, M.L. (1993). The role of body image in sexually avoidant behavior. *Archives of Sexual Behavior, 22*, 345–356.

Fonatana, B. (1994). Plastic sex and the sociologist: A comment on "The transformation of intimacy" by Anthony Giddens. *Economy & Society, 73*, 374–384.

Fooken, L. (1994). Sexuality in later years: The impact of health and body image in a sample of older women. *Patient Education and Counseling, 23*, 227–233.

Foucault, M. (1978). *The History of Sexuality (Part 1): An Introduction.* New York: Random House.

Frank, E., Anderson, C., and Rubinstein, D. (1978). Frequency of sexual dysfunction in "normal" couples. *New England Journal of Medicine, 229*, 111–115.

Geison, C.B. (1989). Aging and attractiveness: Marriage makes a difference. *International Journal of Aging and Human Development, 29*(2), 83–94.

George, L.K., and Weiler, S.J. (1981). Sexuality in middle and late life. *Archives of General Psychiatry, 38*, 919–923.

Hallstrom, T. (1977). Sexuality in the climacteric. *Clinical Obstetrical Gynecology, 4*, 227–239.

Hallstrom, T., and Samuelson, S. (1990). Changes in women's sexual desire in middle life: The longitudinal study of women in Gotenborg. *Archives of Sexual Behavior, 19*, 259–268.

Harris, G. (2004, February 28). Pfizer gives up trying to prove Viagra works for women. *New York Times*, pp. B1, B2.

Irvine, J. (1990). *Disorders of Desire: Sex and Gender in Modern American Sexology.* Philadelphia: Temple University Press.

Kaschak, E., and Tiefer, L. (Eds.). (2001). *A New View of Women's Sexual Problems.* Binghamton, NY: Haworth Press.

Kinsey, A.C., Pomeroy, W.B., and Martin, C.E. (1953). *Sexual Behavior in the Human Female.* Philadelphia: Saunders.

Kliger, L., and Nedelman, D. (2005, July). *Redefining "Sexy": Sexual Desire and Sexual Self-esteem in Women Beyond 50.* Paper presented at the New View Conference, Montreal, Canada.

Kliger, L., and Nedelman, D. (2006). *Still Sexy after all these Years? The 9 Unspoken Truths about Women's Desire.* New York: Berkeley.

Koch, P.B. (1995). *Exploring our Sexuality: An Interactive Text.* Dubuque, IA: Kendall/Hunt.

Koch, P.B. (1997). Feminism and sexuality in the United States. In R.T. Francoeur (Ed.), *The International Encyclopedia of Sexuality* (Vol. 3, pp. 1375–1382). New York: Continuum.

Koch, P.B., Mansfield, P.K., Thurau, D., and Carey, M. (2005). "Feeling frumpy": The relationship between body image and sexual response changes in midlife women. *Journal of Sex Research, 42*, 215–222.

Koch, P.B., Voda, A., and Mansfield, P.K. (1995). Predictors of sexual response changes in heterosexual midlife women. *Health Values, 19*(1), 10–21.

Laumann, E.O., Paik, A., and Rosen, R.C. (1999). Sexual dysfunction in the United States: Prevalence and predictors. *Journal of the American Medical Association, 28*, 537–544.

Laws, J.L. (1980). Female sexuality through the life span. In P.B. Baltes and O.G. Brim, Jr. (Eds.), *Life Span Development and Behavior* (Vol. 3, pp. 207–252). New York: Academic Press.

Leiblum, S.R. (1990). Sexuality and the midlife woman. *Psychology of Women Quarterly, 14*, 495–508.

Leiblum, S.R., and Perrin, L. (Eds.). (1980). *Principles and Practice of Sex Therapy*. New York: Guilford.

Loe, M. (2004). Sex and the senior woman: Pleasure and danger in the Viagra era. *Sexualities, 7*, 303–326.

Mansfield, P.K., Koch, P.B., and Voda, A.M. (1998). Qualities midlife women desire in their sexual relationships and their changing sexual response. *Psychology of Women Quarterly, 22*, 285–303.

Mansfield, P.K., Koch, P.B., and Voda, A.M. (2000). Midlife women's attributions for their sexual response changes. *Health Care for Women International, 31*, 543–559.

Mansfield, P.K., Voda, A.M., and Koch, P.B. (1995). Predictors of sexual response changes in heterosexual midlife women. *Health Values, 19*(1), 10–20.

Marrow, J. (1997). *Changing Positions: Women Speak Out on Sex and Desire*. Holbrook, MA: Adams Media.

Martin, K.A. (1996). *Puberty, Sexuality, and the Self: Girls and Boys at Adolescence*. New York: Routledge.

Masters, W.H., and Johnson, V.E. (1966). *Human Sexual Response*. Boston: Little, Brown.

McCoy, N., Cutler, W.B., and Davidson, J.M. (1985). Relationships among sexual behavior, hot flashes, and hormone levels in peri-menopausal women. *Archives of Sexual Behavior, 14*, 381–390.

McCoy, N.L., and Davidson, J.M. (1985). A longitudinal study of the effects of menopause on sexuality. *Maturitas, 7*, 203–210.

McHugh, M.C. (in press). What do women want? A New View of women's sexual problems. *Sex Roles*.

Miller, J.B. (1976). *Toward a New Psychology of Women*. Boston, MA: Beacon Press.

Morokoff, P.J. (1988). Sexuality in peri-menopausal and post-menopausal women. *Psychology of Women Quarterly, 12*, 489–511.

Moynihan, R. (2001). The making of a disease: Female sexual dysfunction. *British Medical Journal, 326*, 45–57.

Moynihan, R. (2004). Fix for low sex drive puts reporters in a bad patch. *British Medical Journal, 329*, 1294.

Myers, L.S. (1995). Methodological review and meta-analysis of sexuality and menopause research. *Neuroscience and Bio-behavioral Reviews, 19*, 331–314.

Ogden, G. (1999). *Women Who Love Sex: An Inquiry into the Expanding Spirit of Women's Erotic Experience* (rev. ed.). Cambridge, MA: Womanspirit Press.

Osborn, M., Hawton, K., and Gath, D. (1988). Sexual dysfunction among middle-aged women in the community. *British Medical Journal, 296*, 959–962.

Peplau, L.A., and Gordon, S.L. (1985). Women and men in love: Gender differences in close heterosexual relationships. In V.E. O'Leary, R.K. Unger, and B.S. Walston (Eds.), *Women, Gender, and Social Psychology* (pp. 257–291). Hillsdale, NJ: Erlbaum.

Pfeiffer, E., Verwoerdt, A., and Davis, G. (1972). Sexual behavior in middle life. *American Journal of Psychiatry, 128*, 1262–1267.

Potts, A., Gavey, N., Grace, V.M., and Vares, T. (2003) The downside of Viagra: Women's experiences and concerns. *Sociology of Health and Illness, 25*, 697–719.

Richgels, P.B. (1992). Hypoactive sexual desire in heterosexual women: A feminist analysis. *Women & Therapy, 12*(1/2), 123–135.

Riley, A., and Riley, E. (2000). Behavioral and clinical findings in couples where the man presents with erectile disorder: A retrospective study. *International Journal of Clinical Practice, 54*, 220–224.

Shah, S. (2001). The orgasm industry. *Progressive, 65*, 29.

Sheehy, G. (2006). *Sex and the Seasoned Woman: Pursuing the Passionate Life*. New York: Random House.

Schwartz, P., and Rutter, V. (2000). *The Gender of Sexuality*. New York: Rowan & Littlefield.

Taylor, D., and Sumrall, A.C. (1993). *The Time of Our Lives: Women Write on Sex after 40*. Freedom, CA: Crossing Press.

Tiefer, L. (2001a). A new view of women's sexual problems: Why new? Why now? *Journal of Sexual Research, 38*, 89–96.

Tiefer, L. (2001b). Arriving at a "new view" of women's sexual problems: Background, theory, and activism. In E. Kaschak and L. Tiefer (Eds.), *A New View of Women's Sexual Problems* (pp. 63–90). Binghamton, NY: Haworth Press.

Tiefer, L. (1995). *Sex Is not a Natural Act and Other Essays*. Boulder, CO: Westview Press.

Tiggerman, M., and Lynch, J.E. (2002). Body image across the life span in adult women: The role of objectification. *Developmental Psychology, 37*, 243–253.

Tolman, D.L. (2001). Echoes of sexual objectification: Listening for one girl's erotic voice. In D.L. Tolman and M. Brydon-Miller (Eds.), *From Subjects to Subjectivities: A Handbook of Interpretive and Participatory Methods* (pp. 130–144). New York: New York University Press.

Tolman, D.L. (2002). Female adolescent sexuality: An argument for a developmental perspective on the new view of sexual problems. In E. Kaschak and L. Tiefer (Eds.), *A New View of Women's Sexual Problems* (pp. 195–210). Binghamton, NY: Haworth Press.

Trafford, A. (1995, May 16). What the pill did. *Washington Post*. p. 26.

Traupmann, J., Eckles, E., and Hatfield, E. (1982). Intimacy in older women's lives. *Gerontologist, 22*, 493–498.

Vance, C.S. (1984). Pleasure and danger: Toward a politics of sexuality. In C.S. Vance (Ed.), *Pleasure and Danger: Exploring Female Sexuality* (pp. 1–27). Boston: Routledge & Kegan Paul.

Voda, A.M., and George, T. (1986). Menopause. In H.H. Wesley, J.J. Fitzpatrick, and R.L. Taunton (Eds.), *Annual Review of Nursing Research* (pp. 55–75). New York: Springer.

Williams, S.P. (2001). Reaching the hard to reach: Implications of the new view of women's sexual problems. In E. Kaschak and L. Tiefer (Eds.), *A New View of Women's Sexual Problems* (pp. 39–42). Binghamton, NY: Haworth Press.

Winterich, J.A. (2003). Sex, menopause, and culture: Sexual orientation and the meaning of menopause for women's sex lives. *Gender & Society, 17*, 627–642.

Wood, J.M., Mansfield, P.K., and Koch, P. (in press). Negotiating sexual agency: Postmenopausal women's meaning and experiences of sexual desire. *Qualitative Health Research*.

Working Group on Women's Sexual Problems. (n.d.). The "New View" Manifesto. Retreived May 10, 2004 from the Female Sexual Dysfucntion-Alert website: http//www.fsd-alert.org/manifesto.html.

3
Living Longer, Healthier Lives

Susan D. Lonborg and Cheryl B. Travis

Contrary to popular images that portray a bleak future, important life tasks and accomplishments characterize the lives of older women. Midlife women are more likely than not to work full-time, and some will earn the highest salaries of their careers. A high percentage of women in public service or elected office are in their 50s and 60s. Bernadine Healy was in her late 40s when she became the first woman to serve as Director of the National Institutes of Health and later became Director of the American Red Cross. Diane Feinstein was in her late 50s when she was the first woman elected to the U.S. Senate from California; she has subsequently served three terms. Women beyond menopause energize the planning of community parks and greenways projects and serve on school boards. Increasingly older women are likely to run a small business and to provide jobs and paychecks for others. Older women support daughters and sons in transition to adult identities, and, not infrequently, rear their own grandchildren when their adult children suffer illness or economic reversals. Older women have developmental tasks involving their own generativity, values, and significant relationships. They write textbooks, learn new languages, and become articulate advocates for causes of all sorts. These examples of active, vital women run counter to common stereotypes of older women. Therefore, the purposes of this chapter are to examine major findings concerning the health status of women in their 50s and 60s and to explore the health challenges and opportunities this population may experience. Given societal notions about menopausal women, we begin our discussion with the menopausal transition.

Menopause Stereotypes and Estrogen Solutions

Despite the general pattern of productivity among older women and the experience of coming into one's own, media images of older women tend to be negative (Rostosky & Travis, 1996, 2000; Travis, 1993). These cultural messages collectively treat women as different or "Other" (Hare-Mustin & Marecek, 1988; Memmi, 1965). Women are seen as obscure, mysterious, unpredictable, and potentially dangerous. In an implied contrast with men, who are seen as normal and rational, women are understood to be "naturally" more closely tied to their biology. Such a cultural understanding leads readily to the idea that women, their experience, emotions, and behaviors, are best understood in terms of biology, especially reproductive biology. As women age, it is women's flagging biology that is perceived as the problem, and this perception provides a cultural context that supports hormone replacement and estrogen supplements. Popular books and magazine articles promised women they could be "feminine forever," if only they retained their essential biological profile. Thus, a ready "cure" for the negative stereotypic aspects of menopause has traditionally involved replacement of reproductive hormones, particularly estrogens (Chrisler et al., 1991).

Early reports about the health benefits derived from estrogen replacement often were based on self-selected women who sought out treatment and on women who were initially healthier than women who did not seek hormones as preventive medical care. Because participants in these studies differed initially on important health status indicators, later findings that they continued to experience different health outcomes cannot be attributed to hormone replacement. One large-scale study (Luoto et al., 2000) showed no differences in the incidence of acute myocardial infarction (i.e., heart attack) between women using estrogen and those who had never used estrogen supplements. The same study revealed that hopes that estrogen might protect aging women against brain atrophy were unfounded.

Heart Health and Estrogen

The Women's Health Initiative Hormone Replacement Therapy Trial cast an even more skeptical view of the benefits of hormone replacement. The Women's Health Initiative of the National Institutes of Health (launched in 1991 under the leadership of the Director, Bernadine Healy) targeted the prevention of heart disease as a major objective. The 15-year program involved clinical trials to examine, among other questions, the effects of hormone replacement therapy. Recruitment of women into the clinical trial began in 1993 and continued through July 1998. One thought was that women with preexisting heart problems might be a group especially likely to benefit from estrogen interventions. Preliminary reports from this large-scale randomized clinical trial surprised researchers because there was a threefold increase in venous embolisms (i.e., blood clots) among women with preexisting heart disease who were taking hormone replacement (Rossouw, 1999). The study remained in operation for another 3 years, but was stopped in July 2002 because women receiving hormone replacement continued to have notably more cardiac and stroke events than did women in the control arm of the trial. Another arm of the trial involved only women who did not have preexisting heart problems and who were initially healthy at the beginning of the study. This arm of the study was stopped in 2004 when it became apparent that healthy women with no prior heart condition received no benefit. The National Heart Lung and Blood Institute concluded that estrogen plus progestin should NOT be used to prevent heart disease; it has no benefit in preventing heart disease and increases the risk of breast cancer and blood clots. Women with preexisting heart conditions also should not use estrogen plus progestin replacement; it increases the risk of heart attack and blood clots. (Summaries of these reports are available on the web from the National Heart Lung and Blood Institute of NIH at http://www.nhlbi.nih.gov/resources/docs/w-health.htm.)

Breast Cancer and Estrogen

The Women's Health Initiative monitored thousands of women administered hormone replacement involving estrogens and progestin. This study focused on 16,000 women over 50 who were followed for 5 years. The group receiving replacement hormones had nearly a 25% greater risk of developing breast cancer; these cancers were more likely to be larger and more invasive than cancers detected among women taking placebos (Chlebowski et al., 2003). Related reports are consistent in identifying hormone replacement as increasing the risk of breast cancer (McPherson, 2004; Million Women Study Collaborators, 2003; Writing Group for the Women's Health Initiative Investigators, 2002). It is frustrating and infuriating that 25 years ago evidence confirmed just such a risk between estrogen replacement and uterine cancer and suggested that a similar risk existed for breast cancer (Jick et al., 1980; Mack et al., 1976). Yet an entire generation of women was encouraged to pursue estrogen regimens that surely contributed to the incidence of cancer and death. Perhaps even more troubling is the observation that many physicians and researchers today are still looking for ways to continue hormone replacement therapy "safely." More specifically, they suggest that a significant problem with the Women's Health Initiative research was that the women sampled were too old; that is, they should have started hormone therapy earlier in their lives. The question remains: How many more women must die prematurely before this dangerous treatment is finally stopped?

Heart Disease

Most people believe the cultural stereotype that heart disease is a man's disease. However, heart disease is the leading cause of death for women as well as for men in Western societies. For example, in 1995, over 300,000 women were hospitalized specifically for acute myocardial infarction, and over 1.5 million women were hospitalized for chronic ischemic heart disease. In fact, for well over a decade the total number of women hospitalized with some type of cardiovascular condition has been consistently greater than the number of men. This gender pattern has been documented annually from 1990 through 2000 in the National Hospital Discharge Survey conducted by the National Center for Health Statistics (Travis, 2005).

Women in general do not worry as much about heart disease as they do about breast cancer, though heart disease kills many more women. Furthermore, many women have been guided by physicians' beliefs and assumptions that whatever risk they have of heart disease could be handled by estrogen replacement therapy after menopause.

Gender and Treatment

Although heart disease is the leading cause of death among women in the United States, most of the 5.7 million procedures on the heart recorded in 1998 were performed on men. Access to care, diagnostic strategies, and preferred treatments also appear to differ markedly by gender (Healy, 1991; Travis et al., 1993; Wenger, 1985, 1987). A number of studies suggest that these gender patterns are the result of biased decision making. Tobin et al. (1987) reported that abnormal diagnostic findings in nuclear exercise testing resulted in significantly more referrals for cardiac catheterization for men than for women with similar abnormal signs. Another study indicated that women in selected Maryland and Massachusetts hospitals were less likely to undergo diagnostic angiography or coronary artery revascularization than were men (Ayanian & Epstein, 1991) A similar study of patients enrolled in the Survival and Ventricular Enlargement Study for the years 1987 to 1990 (1842 men, 389 women) showed that the health care history of women prior to the initial myocardial infarction indicated a less aggressive management approach than that observed for men (Steingart et al., 1996).

But aren't "things different now"? As a partial answer to this question, detailed records of patients' diagnoses and procedures were examined for trends over the 12-year period from 1987 to 1998. Coronary artery bypass graft (commonly known as bypass surgery or CABG) is one marker by which to track issues of the quality of care and medical decision making with respect to gender. The most frequent and key diagnostic conditions associated with bypass surgery are chronic or acute ischemia (i.e., restriction or shortage of blood supply), angina, and acute myocardial infarction. As diagnostic and surgical methods have become more widely available, bypass surgery has been increasingly viewed as useful, and treatment of heart disease has become more aggressive. This is particularly true for male patients.

There has never been a particularly aggressive or active surgical approach to heart disease if the patient is female, even when women's medical conditions are similar to those of men who receive surgical treatment. Approximately 600,000 bypass surgeries were performed in the United States in 2002, an increase of about 83% over the number performed a decade earlier. The vast majority of those were performed on men. Among patients with key diagnoses, over 50% of men versus only 27% of women had bypass surgery (Travis, 2006).

A number of factors might explain why women tend not to receive bypass surgery. One possibility is that women are older, and physicians and family members may think that there is less potential benefit from aggressive treatment. Of course, if this were the case, then age would be a covariate for procedures performed on men as well as on women. Other explanations might lie in the possibility that women have more preexisting health conditions (e.g., diabetes) that could complicate surgery. Statistical analysis of approximately 10 million patient records over a decade indicated that factors such as older age or comorbid conditions did not account for gender differences. Overall, men were twice as likely to have bypass surgery as were women with comparable medical profiles. This result was particularly evident for women in relatively young age groups (40s and 50s), when angina was a primary diagnosis, and in the presence of any chronic health condition (e.g., diabetes or hypertension) (Travis, 2005). Thus, gender stereotypes and sex discrimination continue to affect decisions about the treatment of midlife and older women with cardiovascular conditions.

Breast Cancer

Cancer is overall the second leading cause of death among women of all ages, and it accounts for nearly one-quarter of deaths from all causes. However, among women 45 to 75 years, it is the leading cause of death (American Cancer Society, 2005). Although it was once rare among women, lung cancer is now one of the more common forms of cancer among women of all ages. Roughly 80,000 U.S. women are diagnosed with lung cancer each year, and nearly an equal number of women die of lung cancer each year (American Cancer Society, 2005). Most of these cases are caused by cigarette smoking, as about 20% of American women smoke (American Cancer Society, 2005; Wolberg, 2004). Notably, rates of cancer vary among White women and Women of Color. Rates of death for all types of cancer are consistently and dramatically higher among Black women than among other race—sex groups (American Cancer Society, 2005).

Although deaths from lung cancer are the most common form of cancer among women, the most dreaded form surely is breast cancer. Approximately 200,000 women are diagnosed with breast cancer each year (American Cancer Society, 2005). Fortunately, about 60% of these cases are detected early, when the tumors are fairly small and localized or in situ (i.e., no involvement of other types of tissues, organs, or lymph nodes). When breast cancer is detected and treated at this early point, 10-year survival rates are very high; estimates range from 72 to 92% (Fletcher et al., 2005; Romero et al., 2004; Solin et al., 2005). As with most major diseases, age is the biggest risk factor for cancer, thus annual mammograms after age 50 are one of the best forms of prevention. Another factor is family history. However, inherited genetic risk accounts for only about 3 to 5% of all breast cancers (Eccles & Pichert, 2005). Short of a genetic screening test, the best indicator of an inherited gene problem is early age of onset. Heritable breast cancers often emerge before women reach menopause, whereas onset at an older age, by itself, conveys little definite information about genetic factors. Thus, having a family member who developed breast cancer at age 75 is not a strong indicator of an inherited genetic problem.

Beyond risks associated with the general processes of aging, a major risk factor for breast cancer is the lifetime exposure to estrogens; the more estrogen, the more breast cancer. It has long been known, for example, that women are at greater risk for breast cancer if they have experienced an early start to menstruation (first menses before age 13) or if they have late menopause (after age 50) (McPherson, 2004). In addition, direct prospective evidence exists for a positive link between levels of estrone and estradiol (forms of estrogen) (Toniolo et al., 1995). Replacement estrogens during menopause are an example of this, and have already been discussed. The potential cancer risk from exogenous estrogens during the years of normal menstrual cycling (ages 13 to 50) is difficult to assess, as virtually all women are also producing their own estrogens at the time.

Coping with Breast Cancer

There are several dimensions and styles of coping; broadly these are social, behavioral, emotional, and cognitive. Women should not feel constrained to adhere solely to one style; the more important consideration is to do what works for the individual woman in her particular circumstances. Social support and interpersonal relations play an important role in coping with any major life stressor, and research has shown that talking about a negative experience tends to reduce overall anxiety and also tends to reduce anxiety responses during future exposures (Lepore et al., 2000).

Behavioral and instrumental coping can include learning more about treatment options, developing patient–physician interaction skills, building relaxation skills, adhering to a general wellness lifestyle for diet and exercise, and practicing good sleep management skills. In consultation with an oncologist and family members, cancer patients typically make a number of decisions about treatment. Depending on the stage of breast cancer, there may be decisions following surgery about whether or not to pursue chemotherapy, radiation therapy, or some combination. Once primary treatments are completed, patients additionally may have the choice whether or not to pursue adjuvant drug therapy, and, if so, the type of drug intervention to be used. Coming to a physician visit prepared to ask specific questions and prepared to negotiate differences of judgment about treatment may foster a greater overall sense of competence for the woman and more equanimity about eventual outcomes and side effects of treatment (Jahng et al., 2005).

Styles of coping may also vary with respect to emotion. For example, some women experience and express anger, anxiety, or grief, whereas other women reduce their emotional responsiveness. One should remember that coping and adjustment evolve and develop with the course of disease and treatment; variation in emotional expressiveness may be useful and appropriate at different times. Managing beliefs and cognitions is another dimension of coping. Some women may actively work at maintaining positive beliefs and thoughts about their treatment, for example, by generating self-labels such as "survivor." However, arbitrarily applying a label such as "survivor" may function to silence some women by forcing them to deny continuing struggles and inner uncertainty. Cognitive coping strategies frequently limit intrusive negative thoughts and avoid catastrophizing. A belief system that characterizes the impact of cancer as comprehensive and permanent may contribute to a sense of helplessness and depression (Barnefski et al., 2002), whereas taking things one step at a time may help to contain negative thoughts and emotions.

Bone and Joint Disease

In addition to cardiovascular disease and cancer, women may experience a number of other chronic conditions; among the most common are diabetes, bone and joint disease, asthma and other breathing-related illnesses, gastrointestinal disorders, and immune system disorders. Each of these illnesses has the potential to alter the quality of women's lives in the fifth and sixth decades; although all are important, we focus here on bone and joint disease.

Bone is a living tissue, which is continuously built and reabsorbed. Cancellous bone is found in the wrist and spine and has a fairly rapid rate of turnover, whereas cortical bone is located in the arms and legs and has a slower rate of cell activity. As they age, many women suffer from a number of potentially debilitating joint diseases; among the most common are osteoporosis and arthritis. Osteoporosis is a skeletal disease characterized by low bone mass and increased porosity of bone tissue (Centers for Disease Control and Prevention, 2005a), whereas the term "arthritis" actually refers to a collection of more than 100 different inflammatory diseases that affect the joints and surrounding connective tissue (Arthritis Foundation, 2005).

Osteoporosis

Eighty percent of individuals in the United States diagnosed with osteoporosis are women; currently at least 10 million Americans have this disease, and another 34 million are at risk for developing it by virtue of their low bone mass (Office of the Surgeon General, 2004). The fact that osteoporosis is the source of the greatest number of fractures in the elderly is perhaps the most health-impairing aspect of this disease. Unfortunately, osteoporosis is both underdiagnosed and undertreated, even in those women who have already suffered at least one fracture. According to the Surgeon General, about 1.5 million people a year suffer an osteoporosis-related fracture, most often in the hip, spine, or wrist; of those with hip fractures, 20% will likely die within a year, and another 20% will end up confined to a nursing home (Office of the Surgeon General, 2004). Clearly, women in their 50s and 60s may benefit not only from early screening, diagnosis, and treatment, but also from health promotion behaviors initiated earlier in their lives. Women are encouraged to ensure that they routinely obtain the recommended amounts of calcium in their diets, engage in a regular program of weight-bearing activity, and request osteoporosis screening (i.e., bone density tests) following any bone fracture. Unfortunately, recent research suggests that strikingly few—18%—of female Medicare patients over age 67 receive either bone density screening or medication following diagnosis of a fracture, despite the fact that treatment of osteoporosis significantly reduces the risk of subsequent fractures (Office of the Surgeon General, 2004). Though it is possible that many older men with fragility fractures do not receive postfracture screening for osteoporosis (Kiebzak et al., 2002), we cannot help but wonder whether health care practitioners would fail to provide the gold standard of care for fractures in older adults (Gardner et al., 2002; Hajcsar et al., 2000) if osteoporosis were a condition diagnosed more often in men rather than in women.

Bone density can be measured, but testing with the most reliable equipment is expensive. Health fairs often offer ultrasound imaging of the heel that produces a quick score, but it is not particularly accurate. Dual X-ray absorptometry (DXA) is the most accurate test. DXA involves a large machine that uses two X-ray beams that are passed through the bone, and typically focuses on the spine and/or hip.

Calcium intake and physical activity throughout life are recommended to prevent osteoporosis. The National Institute of Health Consensus Panel on Calcium concluded that a daily intake of 1500 mg of calcium is recommended for older women, but this intake is seldom met (National Consensus Development Panel on Optimal Calcium Intake, 1994). Natural food sources high in calcium include most dairy products that often are restricted in efforts to control weight or cholesterol. Dark green vegetables typically contain notable levels of calcium; less commonly recognized sources include fruits such as cantaloupes, dried fruits, and many berries. Nutritional supplements of calcium are widely available, but the plethora of formulations can be puzzling. For example, although calcium in the form of carbonate and citrate is absorbed at about the same rate, calcium citrate may be better for people with reduced stomach acid (Office of Dietary Supplements, 2006). Prescription supplements have gained increasing recognition in recent years. Some of the commonly prescribed bisphosphonates are risedronate (Actonel®), alendronate (Fosamax®), and etidronate (Didrocal®). Most of these block the action of osteoclasts that breakdown bone for resorption. Alternative pharmaceutical approaches may use SERMs (special estrogen receptor modulators); side effects associated with SERMs seem to mimic those of menopause, such as hot flashes. Low bone density is associated with more fractures, but the extent to which fracture risk is causally reduced by these pharmaceutical interventions remains to be determined. For example, surveys might indicate a greatly reduced risk of fracture among those taking the medication, even though the medication raised actual bone density only slightly. Whether these studies suffer from the same flaws as the early estrogen replacement studies is, of course, a concern. Women who seek care and follow prescription regimens simply may have better overall health, diet, and lifestyle than those who do not. Thus, the beneficial outcomes of lower fracture may be due as much to lifestyle health as to prescription medications.

Arthritis

Joint diseases constitute the leading cause of disability among American adults and, unfortunately, arthritis rates also increase with age. The rate of arthritis among women age 75 and older is more than five times the rate in women 18 to 44 years of age (National Center for Health Statistics, 2003). Among the most common forms of arthritis are osteoarthritis, rheumatoid arthritis, systemic lupus erythematosus, gout, and fibromyalgia (Centers for Disease Control and Prevention, 2005b). Of these joint diseases, only gout is diagnosed less frequently in women than in men.

Arthritis represents a significant health issue for women in that it is the leading reason for activity limitations in this population (Centers for Disease Control and Prevention, 2005b). Osteoarthritis, characterized by pain and restricted movement occurs most frequently in the knees, hips, spine, and hand. About one-half of all women over the age of 65 experience some pain and some activity limitations associated with this condition (National Center for Health Statistics, 2003). In contrast to the localized nature of osteoarthritis, rheumatoid arthritis is a systemic inflammatory joint disease most likely caused by a faulty immune response. In addition to eroding bone and cartilage, which causes pain, swelling, and redness in the joints, this inflammatory process can also affect other organs. Patients coping with arthritis conditions have a variety of medical and behavioral treatment strategies available to them. Numerous prescription and nonprescription medicines may be used to treat the pain and inflammation associated with these conditions; however, it is important to note that pharmacotherapy is not without side effects or risks. Patients with advanced osteoarthritis may wish to consider joint replacement surgery. Although arthritis-associated pain is often a barrier to exercise, women often find low-impact activities (e.g., water aerobics, swimming) to be both physically tolerable and health enhancing methods of coping with a chronic musculoskeletal condition. Along with exercise, weight management is also essential for reducing stress on weight-bearing joints.

Brain Health and Alzheimer's Disease

Fortunately, the brain is a highly adaptive piece of equipment. Not only is it the command center for motor, sensory, and cognitive functions, it has the capacity to modify or reorganize itself; cortical circuits can be repaired, and new networks of circuits can be integrated, to allow modified function in response to many different traumas. There are things that women can do to enhance or maintain their brain health. Exercise has been found in animal studies to increase the number of tiny blood vessels in the brain, the number of synaptic connections, and even the development of new neurons (Kramer et al., 1999; van Praag et al., 1999). This means that the brain is more efficient, plastic, and adaptive in the context of physical activity. There seem to be differences in the prefrontal and frontal brain regions of physically fit versus unfit humans, and recent clinical trials with humans have shown that problem solving and focused attention are both improved by exercise (Colcombe et al., 2004). Maintaining general physical fitness and daily aerobic exercise are the two best ways to keep brain plasticity and health. In addition, there is some evidence that reducing low-density cholesterol may promote better circulation to the brain and slow cognitive decline (Jick et al., 2000). One way to reduce cholesterol is to reduce the intake of trans or hydrogenated fats (e.g., fried food, prepared snack cakes) and to increase the intake of foods with polyunsaturated, unhydrogenated fats that contain omega essential fatty acids, such as unsaturated vegetable oils (Morris et al., 2003). To this end, the old maxim that fish is brain food may not be far from the truth. Another old saying—"use it or lose it"—also may be pertinent to the maintenance of sharp cognitive function. Social stimulation and interaction is one way to keep cognitive functions active, but this may be difficult for older people with limited mobility whose older friends also have limited mobility. Although heart health has been widely adopted as an important goal of lifestyle behaviors, the same cannot be said for brain health. Nevertheless, it is important because there are a number of risks to brain health as people age.

Alzheimer's Disease (AD) is one of the more common of several forms of dementia, most of which are characterized by memory impairment, inability to recall or appropriately use words in speech, problems of judgment, and motor impairment. Age is the single greatest risk factor for AD, but it is not limited to the extremely aged and infirm. It usually begins in the 40s and 50s, signaled initially by memory lapses and later substantial impairment of attention and speech and eventual confusion and helplessness. Although lapses of memory or difficulty in finding the right word happen to everyone, for those with AD these lapses interfere with the ability to perform daily functions, such as finding one's toothbrush. Odd or idiosyncratic words may be substituted for the word that cannot be retrieved. In addition poor judgment may lead to impulsive or extravagant behavior, which makes individuals with AD more vulnerable to financial scams. The prevalence of AD in the year 2050 is estimated to be roughly 13 million, nearly triple the number of current cases (Hebert et al., 2003). The functional changes in memory and judgment are the result of structural changes in the brain. These include deterioration of brain synapses, the growth of neurofibrillary tangles (i.e., twisted and super-coiled protein fragments inside brain cells), and the buildup of amyloid plaque around brain cells, synapses, and in brain blood vessels (Gylys et al., 2004; Sayre et al., 2005). However, as with most correlational research, one does not know if amyloid and similar proteins *cause* the problems or instead are *responses* that reflect the brain's efforts to cope with other forms of stress or trauma.

The most general risk factor for AD is age. There appears to be more than one genetic precursor that may contribute to early or to late onset, but genetic inheritance is thought to account for only about one-quarter of AD cases. Because higher levels of aluminum have been found in the brains of patients already diagnosed with AD, there has been some concern that aluminum could be a causal factor. Aluminum is widely present in the environment; common sources include some antiperspirants, processed flour in cake and pancake mixes, and processed cheese. Drinking water is probably the most widely dispersed source of human exposure to aluminum. The National Institute of Environmental Health Sciences (Office of Dietary Supplements, 2006) notes that aluminum is widespread in the environment, and most people intake 30 to 50 mg per day; however, less than 1% of the amount ingested is actually absorbed. Most public concern about aluminum and AD has been focused on cookware or beverage containers. However, beverage containers are usually coated with a polymer that would inhibit such exposure. There may be leeching of aluminum from cookware, but it is most likely to occur in the cooking of high acid foods, such as tomatoes. Less widely noted is the possibility that deficiencies in other trace minerals, such as magnesium and phosphorous, may contribute to increased levels of aluminum. Because magnesium and phosphorous have antioxidant effects that could lower the retention of aluminum, one wellness lifestyle pattern is to insure adequate ingestion of magnesium and phosphorous. Dietary sources of magnesium include whole grains, nuts, and leafy vegetables, whereas sources of phosphorous include fish, poultry, meat, eggs, and milk. Unfortunately, general antioxidants, such as vitamin E, are not prevalent in brain tissue, and it is difficult to make a general prescription in favor of prescription of antioxidants as protection from AD (Vinia et al., 2004).

Coping with Chronic Disease

Women may experience any number of different chronic diseases that can result in chronic pain, impaired mobility, activity limitations, relationship stress, or psychological distress. Clearly, it is important to identify those health promoting and coping strategies that may prove beneficial to women encountering symptoms and consequences of chronic illness. Coping strategies and interventions may be primarily patient-centered or more inclusive of the woman's romantic partner or family system. Patient-centered coping strategies are frequently categorized as one of five types (i.e., emotion-focused coping, problem-focused coping, social support, spiritual coping, and cognitive restructuring or meaning making) (Aldwin & Yancura, 2004), although it is important to note that social support and spiritual coping actually contain elements of both emotion- and problem-focused coping.

Emotion-focused coping strategies are those that involve either expressing emotion or engaging in withdrawal, disengagement, or avoidance. Whereas talking about emotions is often considered a positive coping strategy (Lepore et al., 2000), emotional avoidance and withdrawal strategies most often result in more negative health outcomes (Aldwin & Revenson, 1987) and more distressed moods in patients with chronic disease (Kozora et al., 2005). It is also important to note that the relationship between emotions and health is a complex one; for example, weekly measures of both negative affect and positive affect have been associated with levels of pain in women with chronic pain conditions (Zautra et al., 2005). The same study indicated that women with higher levels of overall positive affect (e.g., determined, active, inspired) tended to report lower levels of pain in subsequent weeks; however, weekly increases in pain and stress were also associated with increased negative affect (e.g., nervous, scared, irritable). In summary, Zautra et al. suggested that high levels of positive affect tend to characterize patients who are more resilient when confronted with both increased pain and interpersonal conflict. In an investigation of positive emotions and health, Richman et al. (2005) found that higher levels of hope and curiosity were associated with a decreased likelihood of having or developing any of three common chronic diseases. They suggested that these positive emotions may have protective effects on health, in contrast to the adverse health behaviors (e.g., smoking, excessive alcohol consumption, decreased physical activity) typically associated with negative emotions, such as anxiety, anger, and depression. In their examination of the associations between socioeconomic status (SES), negative emotions, and physical health, Gallo and Matthews (2003) proposed that low-SES environments are often stressful, thereby reducing individuals' "reserve capacity to manage stress" and increasing their vulnerability to negative cognitions (e.g., pessimism, hopelessness) and emotions (e.g., anxiety, depression, worry). In summary, constructive emotion-focused coping strategies should ideally provide opportunities to identify and experience positive emotions (e.g., determination, hope) and also help women to identify and practice methods of coping with those negative emotions that may occur in the context of chronic illness or pain. Positive emotions are generally an indicator of hope and the resolution of doubt. However, one would not want to demand that women have only positive emotions; so-called negative emotions such as anger can also energize positive actions.

In contrast to emotion-focused coping, problem-focused coping strategies are directed at understanding and solving health-related problems. Typically, these methods of coping involve information gathering and planning, strategies that require some degree of activity on the part of the patient. Problem-focused coping methods, particularly information seeking, have been associated with more positive health outcomes (i.e., slower disease progression, fewer symptoms) and improved health-related quality of life (Ransom et al., 2005). Unfortunately, as women age, their risk for other health-compromising conditions (e.g., heart, respiratory, and joint diseases) may increase; in turn, these chronic health problems can potentially limit their ability to engage in some of the more active forms of problem-focused coping (e.g., exercise, relaxation procedures).

Patients are often encouraged to use social support as a source of coping with illness, however, it is important to note that the relationship between social support and health outcomes is somewhat complicated (Aldwin & Yancura, 2004; DiMatteo, 2004). Several studies suggest that social support from family and friends may boost patients' adherence to treatment via a number of different mechanisms, most notably, by encouraging optimism (Brissette et al., 2002; Symister & Friend, 2003), reducing depression and isolation (Brown et al., 1989; Goodenow et al., 1990; Symister & Friend, 2003), and providing practical (or tangible) assistance (DiMatteo, 2004; Wallston et al., 1983). The results of a recent meta-analysis of the social support and treatment adherence literature indicate that "[f]unctional social support has stronger effects on adherence than does structural social support, suggesting that the mere presence of other people does not matter as much as the quality of relationships with them" (DiMatteo, 2004, p. 212). It is not surprising, then, that health professionals have become increasingly interested in relationship (Badr & Acitelli, 2005; Manne et al., 2006) and family-based coping interventions (Martire et al., 2004). The goals of these system-based interventions are ideally to improve patient health outcomes, reduce illness symptoms, enhance psychological well-being, and provide empathy and support (Martire et al., 2004), yet, to date, there are relatively few empirical investigations of the outcomes of such interventions in comparison to individual patient-oriented approaches. In a review of just 12 family-based intervention studies, Martire et al. (2004) found that five of 12 investigations demonstrated clear advantages associated with social support, most notably in the areas of pain severity, sickness impact, psychosocial adjustment, and communication between patients and their family members. Only one of 12 studies confirmed a clear advantage associated with individually oriented interventions; specifically, rheumatoid arthritis patients reported greater self-efficacy and reduced fatigue when attending a patient education program than when participating in a program that included their partners or spouses (Riemsma et al., 2003).

Although more research on the short- and long-term effects of family-based coping interventions is warranted, one couple-focused group intervention for women with early stage breast cancer suggests a particular advantage to this approach. In a study of 238 women randomly assigned to either a 6-week couple-focused intervention or the usual patient-focused care, researchers found that women who experienced more physical impairment or who rated their partners as unsupportive benefited more from the couple-based program (Manne et al., 2005). Women who participated in the group intervention for couples not only reported significantly less distress at the end of the program, but also appeared to demonstrate a longer-term reduction in symptoms of depression. According to the authors, one advantage of the couples-based intervention may be that it allows the partners to discuss with one another the effects of the disease (i.e., breast cancer) on their relationship and daily life.

Accommodating the Limitations Associated with Chronic Disease

Although the aforementioned individual coping strategies are clearly designed to ameliorate or minimize the negative effects of chronic illness, some women will undoubtedly require environmental accommodations as well. In a recent study of work limitations and accommodations for chronically ill employees, investigators identified three distinct areas for work adjustment: physical work demands, cognitive work demands, and social work demands (Munir et al., 2005). In their survey of 610 supervisors, the authors found that, although depression had the largest impact on all three work demand categories, patients with depression were the least likely to receive a cognitive work adjustment. In contrast, employer work adjustments were readily available to employees whose illnesses (e.g., musculoskeletal conditions) required accommodation of their physical work demands. It is interesting that those patients with chronic illnesses other than musculoskeletal conditions were more likely to experience work limitations due to generic symptoms of illness (e.g., fatigue) than limitations due to disease-specific symptoms, and employers' work adjustments to the cognitive demands of the job were most likely to occur in response to employees' disclosure of illness.

Although individuals with disabilities have a legal right to reasonable accommodations in most public, educational, and employment settings (Americans with Disabilities Act, 1990), one barrier to seeking such accommodations may involve the perceptions of the patients' illness. For example, one qualitative study of young female survivors of hemorrhagic stroke showed that these women often expressed concerns about how they might be perceived by others. More specifically, women in the study were clearly aware that stroke is typically viewed as a disease of old age and that "disabilities worth taking seriously are readily visible" (Stone, 2005, p. 293). Despite the possibility of such misperceptions, women who find themselves in need of disability accommodations should be encouraged to pursue whatever mechanisms are available to improve both their quality of life and personal functioning. Such accommodations might include, but are not limited to, work station adjustments (i.e., ergonomic improvements) and other adaptive equipment, improved accessibility, and schedule modifications that will allow for time and access to required health care. Because women's work lives often contribute to their sense of psychological well-being, as well as their financial stability, women should not be pressured to take early retirement or disability until all avenues of workplace accommodation have been explored.

Informational Support

As mentioned previously, problem-focused coping strategies have been frequently linked to improved health outcomes in women. Information seeking represents one such problem-focused approach to coping. Women who have been diagnosed with chronic diseases or conditions often benefit from access to current information about their conditions and available treatment alternatives. Such information is often found from one of three resources: the woman's own health care provider(s), support groups, and print or electronic media. Women with chronic illness ideally will have the opportunity to develop collaborative working relationships with their treatment providers, an issue to which we will return later in this chapter. Disease or condition-specific support groups often provide another important source of information and social support for patients. Although many communities have health information libraries associated with either their local universities or medical centers, the Internet is rapidly becoming a primary source of health information for patients (Bansil et al., 2006) who are dealing with a wide range of chronic diseases.

Community Resources

Whether women are focused primarily on health promotion and disease prevention or are already having chronic health problems, there are a growing number of community resources available for information, education, and support. In some communities, women may avail themselves of the resources of a local community health library; in others, health information may be obtained from county health departments or health care facilities. Those women who have experience with and access to the Internet can find a plethora of information related to health promotion, disease prevention, and the treatment of acute and chronic illness. For example, both the Centers for Disease Control (CDC) and the National Institutes of Health (NIH) maintain Web sites with links to important health and illness information for consumers as well as for their health care providers. Many organizations concerned with education about and prevention of specific diseases (e.g., arthritis, heart disease) have established websites that provide comprehensive information for newly diagnosed patients and their families. Finally, the Internet is home to many electronic support groups that are often established to provide informational and social support for those diagnosed with specific diseases (e.g., inflammatory bowel disease, breast cancer). Women who enter the name of a specific disease or health topic in an Internet search engine (e.g., Google) are likely to find dozens, if not hundreds, of links to websites with information related to their topic of interest. As information becomes more readily available online, women may encounter conflicting information and recommendations, which requires some structure or strategy for evaluating the accuracy and usefulness of the health care recommendations available to them via this medium. One such strategy might involve gathering information from multiple Internet sources, compiling a list of recommendations, and then discussing this information with health care providers to determine the best course of treatment for the individual woman.

As mentioned previously, informational support is often an important component of problem-focused coping. Women who possess up-to-date, accurate information about their illnesses not only may find themselves more empowered to manage their health or illness, but also to advocate for more collaborative and satisfactory relationships with their health care providers.

Planning and Managing Health Care

Whether concerned about health promotion and prevention or the diagnosis and treatment of acute or chronic disease, women must be prepared to manage effectively their relationships with health care and insurance providers. This can pose a particular challenge for those women who conform to traditional gender role expectations of agreeableness, acquiescence, and passivity; sometimes it is more effective to be insistent, steadfast, and gritty. For example, when receiving yet another wait-and-see recommendation from her doctor, one woman laid down in the waiting room floor and refused to move until her symptoms were properly diagnosed; as it turned out, she had a ruptured appendix.

Patient–Provider Relationships

Beginning in adolescence, women are more likely than men to utilize the health care system (National Center for Health Statistics, 2003). Women ages 45 to 64 average more than eight physician contacts per year compared to about six per year for men. It is not surprising then that a number of researchers have examined women's experiences with health care and health care providers. One nationwide study conducted by the Commonwealth Fund's Commission on Women's Health (2003) indicated that women were twice as likely as men to report negative feelings about the patient–provider relationship. More specifically, 25% of women believed that their physicians "talked down to them," and 17% reported that their physicians suggested that their health problems were "all in their heads." According to a special task force report of the American Medical Association, women are more likely than men to have their symptoms attributed to "overanxiousness"—a psychological problem—even when medical test results suggest the presence of an organic (i.e., physical) problem (Task Force, Ethical and Judicial Affairs, American Medical Association, 1991). Physicians may also tend to underestimate women's (and patients of lower socioeconomic status)[1] understanding of medical terminology as well as their interest in receiving technical information, which results in a gender disparity in the technical complexity and specificity of information given to patients (Sprague-Zones, 1995). It is not surprising, then, that women are more likely than men to change physicians, perhaps in large part due to problems in the patient–provider relationship.

Women over 65 participating in focus groups reported that, although their physical health needs were generally met, a number of areas of the patient–provider relationship might otherwise be improved (Tannenbaum et al., 2003). Among these were women's desire to feel validated as active participants in their health care, the importance of recognizing women's aging-related concerns and anxieties, and the need for greater information sharing and education in the patient–provider relationship. The women who participated in that study were particularly interested in learning more about diet, exercise, and other health maintenance strategies associated with successful aging, yet they believed that time, accessibility, and continuity of care represented significant barriers to obtaining effective health care. More specifically, women suggested that their providers did not always have sufficient time to listen to and address their health care concerns or to provide detailed information about the normal aging process. Although patient satisfaction and patient adherence to medical regimens have been found to be improved by a good patient–provider relationship (Carlson & Skochelak, 1998),[2] the fundamental goal always should be to improve the quality of care patients receive. Positive nonverbal behavior, optimistic talk, and social conversation may contribute to an overall good feeling about the encounter, but they should not substitute for technical competence or for thorough understanding of the patients' symptoms and concerns. Similarly, general sociable conversation should not be used to avoid recognition of or resolution of possible disagreements. Fortunately, effective patient–provider communication has been shown to be associated with improved health outcomes in breast cancer, diabetes, hypertension, and peptic ulcer disease (Kaplan et al., 1989).

---

[1] The similarity of patterns for women in general and for anyone in a lower socioeconomic status supports the point that gender is a status or class variable and not simply a personal attribute.

[2] Research has suggested that female physicians may engage in more interactive question asking and dialogue (Bertakis et al., 1995; Roter et al., 1991). However, this is sometimes confounded with the area of specialization, for example, pediatrics.

Consent to Treatment

Women with acute or chronic disease often face a number of important decisions concerning their treatment. Although advances in technology afford women more opportunity than ever to collect independent information about available treatment alternatives, treatment decisions ultimately develop in the context of an individual patient's relationship with her health care provider. Consequently, informed consent to treatment becomes an issue of paramount importance.

Informed Consent to Treatment

In contrast to the popular view that treatment consent is the signing of a document, informed consent is more accurately viewed as "a process by which a fully informed patient can participate in choices about her health care. It originates from the legal and ethical right the patient has to direct what happens to her body and from the ethical duty of the physician to involve the patient in her health care" (Edwards, 1998, p. 1). The informed consent process should enable women and their health care providers to engage in a collaborative treatment relationship, one that is in direct contrast to the historical conception of paternalistic physicians who independently make decisions that they believe to be in the best interests of their patients.

True informed consent involves a voluntary decision to accept a particular treatment and occurs when a woman is free from coercion or unfair inducements. It is a process of communication and exchange. Medical ethics require that patients be informed about and consent to treatment (American Medical Association, Council on Ethical and Judicial Affairs, 2004; delCarmen & Joffe, 2005). Failure to engage in this process can be considered legally to be battery and/or negligence. A number of specific elements are included in full informed consent; these include the following: (a) receipt of a diagnosis; (b) proposed treatment, goals that the treatment may accomplish, and the likelihood of achieving those goals; (c) potential risks and side effects of the proposed treatment; (d) alternative treatments, regardless of cost, as well as the potential risks and side effects of alternative treatments; and (e) the possibility of doing nothing or waiting, and the problems outcomes of such a course.

Unfortunately, there continue to be gaps between what health care providers believe about informed consent and their actual consent-related behaviors. For example, research on the reading level of informed consent documents included in clinical treatment trials suggests that few informed consent documents are actually written at the average reading level of adults in the United States, that is, the eighth grade level. In fact, nearly one-half of the informed consent forms reviewed required a college level reading ability (Reidenberg, 2005). These data suggest that the mere fact of a patient's signature on an informed consent document does not necessarily imply that she has been fully informed of the treatment to which she has presumably "consented." Fortunately, there is a growing call among health care professionals to view informed consent as a *process* rather than as a form to be signed (King, 2005; Yamalik, 2005) as well as to be mindful of the cultural contexts in which individual patients make decisions (Simon & Kodish, 2005). One might argue, then, that empowering women truly to engage in informed consent for treatment means that, as a society, we must work to ensure that all people, regardless of gender, race, culture, and class have a range of treatment options readily available to them. Similarly, health care providers must create an environment in which patients are invited to ask questions about proposed treatments and treatment alternatives. This is particularly important for those women who, by virtue of gender socialization or education, may be otherwise hesitant to indicate they do not fully understand the information provided to them.

A frequent, but seldom discussed, aspect of informed consent is consent to the involvement of observers or trainees. One common practice, referred to as "shadowing," allows others to observe treatment, for example, during surgery. The observers often are medical interns or residents, and the observation's benefit is to the trainee, not to the patient. If the student, intern, or other paraprofessional is to engage in any examination of the patient or engage in any procedure involving the patient, this should be clarified in advance. Patients should be informed of, and allowed to give or withhold consent, to such observation, and they should receive assurance that the observer has in fact completed appropriate training. Further, consent to allow other unnamed individuals to be involved in treatment should extend only to procedures directly and specifically related to the condition for which the individual is receiving treatment. The possible ways in which this practice may be misused can be surmised from denials issued by hospitals that they have never allowed, or no longer allow, questionable practices to occur as a result of such blanket consent. Observation or shadowing can allow, for example, representatives from pharmaceutical companies to be present during surgery and other treatment; in most instances, such individuals do not have medical training.

Advance Directives

Given the ethical and legal climate in health care today, women are strongly encouraged to anticipate and plan for the possibility that they, at some point in the future, may not be capable of providing informed consent for medical treatment. A number of legal documents have been designed to assist patients in communicating their wishes should such circumstances arise. More specifically, women of all ages—but particularly those in midlife—are advised to prepare advance directives for health care. Generally, three types of advance directives are available: a living will, a durable power of attorney for health care, and a do-not-resuscitate (DNR) order. Such documents are intended to provide patients' families and health care providers with specific instructions about future treatment and to identify those who have been legally authorized to make treatment decisions on behalf of the patient.

One type of written document, the *living will*, describes for family members and health care providers the types of medical care the patient wants to receive in the event of a terminal illness or a permanently unconscious state (Geller, n.d.). Living wills typically take effect at the point at which a physician determines that a patient, because of illness, is unable to communicate decisions about her medical care. In short, the purpose of the living will is to communicate the patient's preferences about what the medical treatment should and should not be. In contrast, the *durable power of attorney for health care* is a written document that describes who is permitted to make decisions on behalf of the patient. In essence, the individual identified as the durable power of attorney for health care becomes an advocate for the patient in the event that the patient, by virtue of illness or injury, becomes cognitively unable to make decisions. One potentially important treatment decision is the use of life-saving medical interventions. Although the living will and durable power of attorney documents provide the legal means for others to make health care decisions for a woman who is incapacitated by illness or injury, end-of-life decisions are often particularly complicated and difficult to make. A patient who does not want to be resuscitated in the event that her breathing and heartbeat stops should be encouraged to document these wishes in writing in a document known as the DNR order.

Although a number of studies indicate that both medical outpatients and inpatients have generally favorable attitudes toward advance directives (Broadwell et al., 1993; Holley et al., 1997; Salmond & David, 2005), relatively few patients actually complete them. Despite the relatively low rates of use of advance directives in the general hospital setting, documents such as the living will, the durable power of attorney for health care, and the DNR order remain important vehicles by which women can communicate to family members, health care providers, and the courts their preferences for medical decision making and treatment.

Taking Charge of Women's Health Care

By now it should be clear that we support a multidimensional view of women's health at midlife. Rather than simply subscribing to a purely biological view of women's health, we make the case that health promotion, disease prevention, and disease management must be understood in the context of the social, cultural, and psychological factors that interact with women's biology in producing various health outcomes. Thus, if we are to identify ways in which women can take care of their own health, we must explore the individual, relational, professional, and societal contexts in which women experience health and illness.

At an individual level, we must continue to support women—particularly older women—in developing the skills to be assertive agents who feel entitled to speak for themselves. The research literature is replete with examples of the ways in which older women have been socialized into submissive positions in relationships with the personal and professional others in their lives (e.g., Weitzman & Weitzman, 2000), which decrease their sense of personal authority and often increase their sense of vulnerability. There is a commonly accepted belief that women are "naturally" inclined and most fulfilled when their actions are guided by the goals of nurturing and caring for others. This orientation has been valorized as a moral framework that is predominate among, if not unique to, women. In fact, a systematic review of research on gender differences in a care perspective of morality indicates that differences are small and that most women and men rely on a combination of attention to principled rules and to relational caring (Jaffe & Hyde, 2000). Although many women may feel guilty about being assertive or advocating for themselves, such agentic behavior may foster better problem solving and greater satisfaction with outcomes. As noted earlier in this chapter, women benefit from a number of health-promoting behaviors (e.g., nutrition, physical activity, stress management), particularly when established earlier in their lives, however, given the multiple role demands often experienced by adult women, it may be difficult to find time for these health-promoting activities. Consequently, we must encourage women to view self-care as a priority in their lives and to implement healthy behaviors in support of that goal. For many women, this is easier said than done, but important nonetheless.

In thinking about ways to support women's health at midlife, we consider both educational and action strategies at four levels: (a) the individual woman; (b) the relationship and family system; (c) the professional health care provider; and (d) society and public policy. For the individual woman, we cannot overstate the importance of education about health-promoting behaviors, disease prevention, and both emotion- and problem-focused approaches to managing chronic health conditions. It is also clear that women often benefit from increased knowledge of their own bodies and health status, as well as from greater personal advocacy when dealing with health care providers and systems.

At a relational or family system level, it is important once again to acknowledge the social context of women's lives. A woman's health may be affected by the circumstances in which she lives; in turn, when women are living with chronic health conditions or pain there are likely to be effects on the family system. For example, research with sheltered homeless and low-income women suggests that physical violence and childhood physical or sexual abuse are associated with avoidant coping strategies and increased depression (Rayburn et al., 2005). In contrast, functional social support from family and friends is often an important contributor to a woman's ability to cope with challenging health conditions. Encouraging family members to become educated about the symptoms, course, and treatment of a disease may improve their understanding of women's experience; similarly, improving communication between women and their intimate partners may help to ameliorate the negative effects of illness and pain on such interpersonal relationships.

Health care providers who work with women at midlife should commit themselves to a number of supportive practices; for example, taking time to provide information to patients, engaging women as collaborators in the health care relationship, and encouraging and supporting informed, autonomous decision-making about the prevention and management of disease. We expect that practitioners would also avail themselves of the current medical and behavioral scientific literature that addresses the health status and health care needs of women at midlife and beyond.

Finally, at a societal level, we advocate for continued research on women's health status and women's experience of chronic illness and disease, with emphasis on understanding the needs of ethnically, culturally, sexually, and economically diverse groups of women. Along with increased knowledge of women's health at midlife, it is also important to improve access to both health promotion resources and health care providers, particularly for those women with limited financial resources. Improvement of access to health care ideally would result in women being more able to make truly informed choices about their health care and treatment. Women who experience chronic conditions or disability should continue to benefit from appropriate accommodations in the workplace and in public facilities.

Despite the challenges to women's health at midlife and continued concerns about gender disparities in health care, women in their 50s today are living longer, healthier lives than their mothers and grandmothers did. They are better educated, more active physically and professionally, and, as a group, have better access to current health care information and resources. As women at midlife support one another in both managing chronic conditions and promoting healthy lifestyles, they also serve as role models for future generations of healthy women. Rather than retiring from life, many older women find opportunity to explore aspects of their lives they previously had not developed. Compared to traditional stereotypes, lifestyles among today's older women are increasingly varied and are more physically active, intellectually expansive, politically effective, socially connected, and healthy.

References

Aldwin, C.M., and Revenson, T.A. (1987). Does coping help? A reexamination of the relation between coping and mental health. *Journal of Personality and Social Psychology, 53*, 337–348.

Aldwin, C.M., and Yancura, L.A. (2004). Coping and health: A comparison of the stress and trauma literature. In P.P. Schnurr and B.L. Green (Eds.), *Physical Health Consequences of Exposure to Extreme Stress* (pp. 99–125). Washington, DC: American Psychological Association.

American Cancer Society. (2005). Estimated new cancer cases and deaths by sex for all sites. *Cancer Facts and Figures*. Retrieved 9-19-05, from http://www.cancer.org/docroot/STT/stt_0.asp:

American Medical Association, Council on Ethical and Judicial Affairs. (2004). *Code of Medical Ethics, Current Opinions with Annotations 2004–2004*. Chicago: American Medical Association.

Americans with Disabilities Act of 1990. (1990). Retrieved 1-12-06, from http://www.usdoj.gov/crt/ada/pubs/ada.txt: U.S. Department of Justice

Arthritis Foundation. (2005). *The Facts about Arthritis*. Retrieved 11/6/05, from http://www.arthritis.org/resources/gettingstarted/default.asp.

Ayanian, J.Z., and Epstein, A.M. (1991). Differences in the use of procedures between women and men hospitalized for coronary heart disease. *New England Journal of Medicine, 325*, 221–225.

Badr, H., and Acitelli, L.K. (2005). Dyadic adjustment in chronic illness: Does relationship talk matter? *Journal of Family Psychology, 19*, 465–469.

Bansil, P., Keenan, N.L., Zlot, A.I., and Gilliland, J.C. (2006). Health-related information on the Web: Results from the Health Styles Survey, 2002–2003. *Preventing Chronic Disease, 3*(2), A36.

Barnefski, N., Legerstee, J., Kraaij, V., van-den Kommer, T., and Teerds, J. (2002). Cognitive coping strategies and symptoms of depression and anxiety: A comparison between adolescents and adults. *Journal of Adolescence, 25*, 603–611.

Bertakis, K.D., Helms, L.J., Callahan, E.J., Azari, R., and Robbins, J.A. (1995). The influence of gender on physician practice style. *Medical Care, 33*, 407–416.

Brissette, I., Scheier, M.F., and Carver, C.S. (2002). The role of optimism in social network development, coping, and psychological adjustment during a life transition. *Journal of Personality and Social Psychology, 82*, 102–111.

Broadwell, A.W., Boisaubin, E.V., Dunn, L.K., and Engelhardt, H.T. (1993). Advance directives on hospital admission: A survey of patient attitudes. *Southern Medical Journal, 86*(2), 165–168.

Brown, G.K., Wallston, K.A., and Nicassio, P.M. (1989). Social support and depression in rheumatoid arthritis: A one-year prospective study. *Journal of Applied Social Psychology, 19*, 1164–1181.

Carlson, K.J., and Skochelak, S.E. (1998). What do women want in a doctor? Communication issues between women and physicians. In L.A. Wallis (Ed.), *Textbook of Women's Health* (pp. 33–38). Philadelphia: Lippincott-Raven.

Centers for Disease Control and Prevention. (2005a). *Bone Health*. Retrieved 11/1/05, from http://www.cdc.gov/needphp/dnpa/bonehealth/: Centers for Disease Control and Prevention.

Centers for Disease Control and Prevention. (2005b). *Arthritis*. Retrieved 11/1/05, from http://www.cdc.gov/arthritis/index.htm: Centers for Disease Control and Prevention

Chlebowski, R.T., Hendrix, S.L., Langer, R.D., Stefanick, M.L., Gass, M., Lane, D., Rodabough, R.J., Gilligan, M.A., Cyr, M.G., Thomson, C.A., Khandekar, J., Petrovitch, H., McTiernan, A., and Women's Health Initiative Investigators. (2003). Influence of estrogen plus progestin on breast cancer and mammography in healthy postmenopausal women: The Women's Health Initiative randomized trial. *Journal of the American Medical Association, 289*, 3243–3253.

Chrisler, J.C., Torrey, J.W., and Matthes, M.M. (1991). Brittle bones and sagging breasts, loss of femininity and loss of sanity: The media describe the menopause. In A.M. Voda and R. Conover (Eds.), *Proceedings of the 8th conference of the Society for Menstrual Cycle Research* (pp. 23–35). Salt Lake City: Society for Menstrual Cycle Research.

Colcombe, S.J., Kramer, A.F., Erickson, K.I., Scalf, P., McAuley, E., Cohen, N.J., Webb, A., Jerome, G.J., Marquez, D.X., and Elavsky, S. (2004). Cardiovascular fitness, cortical plasticity, and aging. *Proceedings of the National Academy of Sciences, 101*, 3316–3321.

Commission on Women's Health. (2003). *The Commonwealth Fund Survey of Women's Health*. New York: Commonwealth Fund.

delCarmen, M.G., and Joffe, S. (2005). Informed consent for medical treatment and research: A review. *Oncologist, 10*, 636–641.

DiMatteo, M.R. (2004). Social support and patient adherence to medical treatment: A meta-analysis. *Health Psychology, 23*, 207–218.

Eccles, D.M., and Pichert, G. (2005). Familial non-BRCA1/BRCA2-associated breast cancer. *Lancet Oncology, 6*, 705–711.

Edwards, K.A. (1998). *Ethics in Medicine: Informed Consent.* Retrieved 11/5/05, from http://depts.washington.edu/bioethx/topics/consent.html.
Fletcher, A.S., Erbas, B., Kavanaugh, A.M., Hart, S., Rodger, A., and Gertig, D.M. (2005). Use of hormone replacement therapy (HRT) and survival following breast cancer diagnosis. *Obstetrical and Gyncological Survey, 60,* 650–651.
Gallo, L.C., and Matthews, K.A. (2003). Understanding the association between socioeconomic status and physical health: Do negative emotions play a role? *Psychological Bulletin, 129,* 10–51.
Gardner, M.J., Flik, K.R., Mooar, P., and Lane, J.M. (2002). Improvement in the undertreatment of osteoporosis following hip fracture. *Journal of Bone and Joint Surgery, 84,* 1342–1348.
Geller, B. (n.d.). *Planning for Medical Care in the Event of Loss of Decision-making Ability.* Retrieved 11/6/05, from http://www.michbar.org/elderlaw/adpamphlet.cfm: Michigan Bar Association.
Goodenow, C., Reisine, S.T., and Grady, K.E. (1990). Quality of social support and associated social and psychological functioning in women with rheumatoid arthritis. *Health Psychology, 9,* 266–284.
Gylys, K.H., Fein, J.A., Yang, F., Wiley, D.J., Miller, C.A., and Cole, G.M. (2004). Synaptic changes in Alzheimer's disease: Increased amyloid and gliosis in surviving terminals is accompanied by decreased PSD-95 fluorescence. *American Journal of Pathology, 165,* 1809–1817.
Hajcsar, E.E., Hawker, G., and Bogoch, E.R. (2000). Investigation and treatment of osteoporosis in patients with fractures. *Canadian Medical Association Journal, 163,* 819–822.
Hare-Mustin, R.T., and Marecek, J. (1988). The meaning of difference: Gender theory, postmodernism, and psychology. *American Psychologist, 43,* 455–464.
Healy, B. (1991). The Yentil syndrome [Editorial]. *New England Journal of Medicine, 325,* 274–276.
Hebert, L.E., Scherr, P.A., Bienias, J.L., Bennett, D.A., and Evans, D.A. (2003). Alzheimer's Disease in the US population: Prevalence estimates using the 2000 census. *Archives of Neurology, 60,* 1119–1122.
Holley, J.L., Stackiewicz, L., Dacko, C., and Rault, R. (1997). Factors influencing dialysis patients' completion of advance directives. *American Journal of Kidney Disease, 30,* 356–360.
Jaffe, S., and Hyde, J.S. (2000). Gender differences in moral orientation: A meta-analysis. *Psychological Bulletin, 126,* 703–726.
Jahng, K.H., Martin, L.R., Golin, C.E., and DiMatteo, M.R. (2005). Preferences for medical collaboration: Patient–physician congruence and patient outcomes. *Patient Education and Counseling, 57,* 308–314.
Jick, H., Walker, A.M., Watkins, R.N., D'Ewart, D.C., Hunter, J.R., Danford, A., Madsen, S., Dinan, B.J., and Rothman, K.J. (1980). Replacement estrogens and breast cancer. *American Journal of Epidemiology, 112,* 586–594.
Jick, H., Zornberg, G.L., Jick, S.S., Seshadri, S., and Drachman, D.A. (2000). Statins and the risk of dementia. *Lancet, 357,* 1627–1631.
Kaplan, S.H., Greenfield, S., and Ware, J.E. (1989). Assessing the effects of physician–patient interactions on the outcomes of chronic disease. *Medical Care, 27,* S110–S127.
Kiebzak, G.M., Beinart, G.A., Perser, K., Ambrose, G.C., Siff, S.J., and Heggeness, M.H. (2002). Undertreatment of osteoporosis in men with hip fracture. *Archives of Internal Medicine, 162,* 2217–2222.

King, J. (2005). Informed consent: Does practice match conviction? *Journal of the American College of Dentists, 72*, 27–31.

Kozora, E., Ellison, M.C., Waxmonsky, J.A., Wamboldt, F.S., and Patterson, T.L. (2005). Major life stress, coping styles, and social support in relation to psychological distress in patients with systemic lupus erythematosus. *Lupus, 14*, 363–372.

Kramer, A.F., Hahn, S., Cohen, N.J., Banich, M.T., McAuley, E., Harrison, C.R., Chason, J., Vakil, E., Bardell, L., Boileau, R.A., and Colcombe, A. (1999). Ageing, fitness, and neurocognitive function. *Nature, 400*, 418–419.

Lepore, S.J., Ragan, J.D., and Jones, S. (2000). Talking facilitates cognitive-emotional processes of adaptation to an acute stressor. *Journal of Personality and Social Psychology, 78*, 499–508.

Luoto, R., Manolio, T., Meilahn, E., Bhadelia, R., Furberg, C., and Cooper, L. (2000). Estrogen replacement therapy and MRI-demonstrated cerebral infarcts, white matter changes, and brain atrophy in older women: The Cardiovascular Health Study. *Journal of the American Geriatrics Society, 48*, 467–472.

Mack, T.N., Pike, M.C., Henderson, B.E., Pfeffer, R.I., Gerkings, V.R., Arthur, M., and Brown, S.E. (1976). Estrogens and endometrial cancer in a retirement community. *New England Journal of Medicine, 294*, 1262–1267.

Manne, S.L., Ostroff, J.S., Norton, T.R., Fox, K., Goldstein, L., and Grana, G. (2006). Cancer-related relationship communication in couples coping with early stage breast cancer. *Psychooncology 15*, 234–247.

Manne, S.L., Ostroff, J.S., Winkel, G., Fox, K., Grana, G., Miller, E., Ross, S., and Frazier, T. (2005). Couple-focused group intervention for women with early stage breast cancer. *Journal of Consulting and Clinical Psychology, 73*, 634–646.

Martire, L.M., Lustig, A.P., Schulz, R., Miller, G.E., and Helgeson, V.S. (2004). Is it beneficial to involve a family member? A meta-analysis of psychosocial interventions for chronic illness. *Health Psychology, 23*, 599–611.

McPherson, K. (2004). Where are we now with hormone replacement therapy? *British Medical Journal, 328*, 357–358.

Memmi, A. (1965). *The Colonizer and the Colonized*. Boston: Beacon Press.

Million Women Study Collaborators. (2003). Breast cancer and hormone-replacement therapy in the Million Women Study. *Lancet, 362*, 419–427.

Morris, M.C., Evans, D.A., Bienias, J.L., Tangney, C.C., Bennett, D.A., Aggarwal, N., Schneider, J., and Wilson, R.S. (2003). Dietary fats and risk of incidents of Alzheimer's Disease. *Archives of Neurology, 60*, 194–200.

Munir, F., Jones, D., Leka, S., and Griffiths, A. (2005). Work limitations and employer adjustments for employees with chronic illness. *International Journal of Rehabilitation, 28*, 111–117.

National Center for Health Statistics. (2003). *National Health Interview Survey*. Atlanta: Centers for Disease Control and Prevention.

National Consensus Development Panel on Optimal Calcium Intake. (1994). NIH consensus conference. Optimal calcium intake. *Journal of the American Medical Association, 272*, 1942–1948.

Office of Dietary Supplements, National Institute of Environmental Health Sciences. (2006). *Dietary Supplement Fact Sheet: Calcium*. In. Retrieved November 21, 2005, from http://ods.od.nih.gov/factsheets/calcium.asp#h10.

Office of the Surgeon General. (2004). *Bone Health and Osteoporosis: A Report of the Surgeon General*. Rockville, MD: U.S. Department of Health and Human Services

Ransom, S., Jacobsen, P.B., Schmidt, J.E., and Andrykowski, M.A. (2005). Relationship of problem-focused coping strategies to changes in quality of life following treatment for early stage breast cancer. *Journal of Pain Symptom Management, 30*, 243–253.

Rayburn, N.R., Wenzel, S.L., Elliott, M.N., Hambarsoomians, K., Marshall, G.N., and Tucker, J.S. (2005). Trauma, depression, coping, and mental health service seeking among impoverished women. *Journal of Consulting and Clinical Psychology, 73*, 667–677.

Reidenberg, M.M. (2005). Informed consent or acknowledgment of disclosure [Letter to the editor]. *Clinical Pharmacology & Therapeutics, 78*, 439–440.

Richman, L.S., Kubzansky, L., Maselko, J., Kawachi, I., Choo, P., and Bauer, M. (2005). Positive emotion and health: Going beyond the negative. *Health Psychology, 24*, 422–429.

Riemsma, R.P., Taal, E., and Rasker, J.J. (2003). Group education for patients with rheumatoid arthritis and their partners. *Arthritis Care and Research, 49*, 556–566.

Romero, L., Klein, L., Ye, W., Holmes, D., Soni, R., Silberman, H., Lagios, M.D., and Silverstein, M.J. (2004). Outcome after invasive recurrence in patients with ductal carcinoma in situ of the breast. *American Journal of Surgery, 188*, 371–376.

Rossouw, J.E. (1999). Hormone replacement therapy and cardiovascular disease. *Current Opinion in Lipidology, 10*, 429–434.

Rostosky, S.C., and Travis, C.B. (1996). Menopause: An examination of the medical and psychological literature 1984–1994. *Psychology of Women Quarterly, 20*, 291–318.

Rostosky, S.S., and Travis, C.B. (2000). Menopause and sexuality: Ageism and sexism unite. In C.B. Travis and J.W. White (Eds.), *Sexuality, Society, and Feminism* (pp. 181–210). Washington, DC: American Psychological Association.

Roter, D., Lipkin, M., and Korsgaard, A. (1991). Sex differences in patients' and physicians' communication during primary care medical visits. *Medical Care, 29*, 1083–1093.

Salmond, S.W., and David, E. (2005). Attitudes toward advance directives and advance directive completion rates. *Orthopedic Nursing, 24*, 117–127.

Sayre, L.M., Moreira, P.I., Smith, M.A., and Perry, G. (2005). Metal ions and oxidative protein modification in neurological disease. *Annals of the Instituto Superiore di Sanità, 41*(2), 143–164.

Simon, C.M., and Kodish, E.D. (2005). "Step into my zapatos, doc": Understanding and reducing communication disparities in the multicultural informed consent setting. *Perspectives in Biology and Medicine, 48*(1), S123–S138.

Solin, L.J., Fourquet, A., Vicini, F.A., Taylor, M., Olivotto, I.A., Haffty, B., Strom, E.A., Pierce, L.J., Marks, L.B., Bartelink, H., McNeese, M.D., Jhingran, A., Wai, E., Bijker, N., Campana, F., and Hwang, W.T. (2005). Long-term outcome after breast-conservation treatment with radiation for mammographically detected ductal carcinoma in situ of the breast. *Cancer, 103*, 1137–1146.

Sprague-Zones, J. (1995). Gender effects in physician/patient interaction. In M. Lipkin, S. Putnam, and A. Lazare (Eds.), *The Medical Interview: Clinical Care, Education, and Research* (pp. 163–171). New York: Springer-Verlag.

Steingart, R.M., Forman, S., Coglianese, M., Bittner, V., Mueller, H., Frishman, W., Handberg, E., Gambino, A., Knatterud, G., and Conti, C.R. (1996). Factors limiting the enrollment of women in a randomized coronary artery disease trial. *Clinical Cardiology, 19*, 614–618.

Stone, S.D. (2005). Reactions to invisible disability: The experiences of young women survivors of hemorrhagic stroke. *Disability Rehabilitation, 27*, 293–304.

Symister, P., and Friend, R. (2003). The influence of social support and problematic support on optimism and pessimism in chronic illness: A prospective study evaluating self-esteem as a mediator. *Health Psychology, 22*, 123–129.

Tannenbaum, C.B., Nasmith, L., and Mayo, N. (2003). Understanding older women's health care concerns: A qualitative study. *Journal of Women and Aging, 15*(4), 103–116.

Task Force, Ethical and Judicial Affairs, American Medical Association. (1991). Gender disparities in clinical decision-making. *Journal of the American Medical Association, 266,* 559–562.

Tobin, J.N., Wassertheil-Smoller, S., Wexler, J.P., Steingard, R.M., Budner, N., Lense, L., and Wachspress, J. (1987). Sex bias in considering coronary bypass surgery. *Annals of Internal Medicine, 107,* 19–25.

Toniolo, P.G., Levitz, M., Zeleniuch-Jacquotte, A., Banerjee, S., Koenig, K.L., Shore, R.E., Strax, P., and Pasternack, B.S. (1995). A prospective study of endogenous estrogens and breast cancer in postmenopausal women. *Journal of the National Cancer Institute, 87*(3), 190–197.

Travis, C.B. (1993, January). *Psychological Aspects of Menopause.* Invited address at the conference on Women's Voices/Women's Bodies: Psychological Aspects of Women's Health, Albuquerque, NM.

Travis, C.B. (2005). Heart disease and gender inequity. *Psychology of Women Quarterly, 29,* 15–23.

Travis, C.B. (2006, March). *Methods to Quantify Gender and Race Disparities.* Paper presented at the meeting of the Southeastern Psychological Association, Atlanta, GA.

Travis, C.B., Gressley, D.L., and Phillippi, R.H. (1993). Medical decision making, gender, and coronary heart disease. *Journal of Women's Health, 2,* 269–279.

van Praag, H., Christie, B.M., Sejnowski, T.J., and Gage, F.H. (1999). Running enhances neurogenesis, learning, and long-term potentiation in mice. *Proceedings of the National Academy of Sciences, 96,* 13427–13431.

Vinia, J., Lloret, A., Orti, R., and Alonso, D. (2004). Molecular bases of the treatment of Alzheimer's disease with antioxidants. *Molecular Aspects of Medicine, 25,* 117–123.

Wallston, B.S., Alagna, S.W., DeVellis, B.M., and DeVellis, R.F. (1983). Social support and physical health. *Health Psychology, 2,* 367–391.

Weitzman, P.F., and Weitzman, E.A. (2000). Interpersonal negotiation strategies in a sample of older women. *Journal of Clinical Geropsychology, 6,* 269–276.

Wenger, N.K. (1985). Coronary disease in women. *Annual Review of Medicine, 36,* 285–294.

Wenger, N.K. (1987). Coronary heart disease in women: Clinical syndromes, prognosis and diagnostic testing. In E.D. Eaker, B. Packard, and N.K. Wenger (Eds.), *Coronary Heart Disease in Women* (pp. 173–186). New York: Haymarket Doyma.

Wolberg, W.H. (2004). *Benign Breast Disease and Breast Cancer Tutorial.* Retrieved September 18, 2005, from http://www.wisc.edu/wolberg/breast.html#endogenous%20estrogen.

Writing Group for the Women's Health Initiative Investigators. (2002). Risks and benefits of estrogen and progestin in healthy postmenopausal women: Principal results from the women's health initiative randomized trial. *Journal of the American Medical Association, 288,* 321–333.

Yamalik, N. (2005). Dentist–patient relationship and quality care: Professional information and informed consent. *International Dentistry Journal, 55,* 342–344.

Zautra, A.J., Johnson, L., and Davis, M.C. (2005). Positive affect as a source of resilience for women in chronic pain. *Journal of Consulting and Clinical Psychology, 73,* 212–220.

4
On the Move: Exercise, Leisure Activities, and Midlife Women

Ruth L. Hall

A few weeks before my 50th birthday, I received a letter from the American Association for Retired People (AARP) informing me that I was now eligible to join AARP. I had arrived. But what did that mean? I'm postmenopausal and beginning to gray more quickly. My physician told me that I had "age-related osteoarthritis," as if that makes the pain any better. Other symptoms of aging continue to emerge. Middle age is a time when our bodies remind us of the process of aging, a time when we say to ourselves, "I don't remember this [body part] giving me trouble when I did [blank] in the past." It is a time to become more active in developing and sustaining a lifestyle that will help us to remain mentally alert, spiritually fulfilled, and physically sound as we grow older.

As a baby boomer, I came of age in the '60s—a time of activism for many oppressed populations throughout the United States and worldwide. The Civil Rights Movement morphed into many other strong movements: the Black Power Movement, the Women's Movement, and the Gay Rights Movement. In some instances, the momentum of the '60s created policies and laws that were concrete signs of progress—Affirmative Action and *Roe v. Wade* altered the landscape for many people. Another legal coup for women in the United States was Title IX, which required federally funded high schools, colleges, and universities to provide equity for girls and women with their male counterparts in sport. All of these legal interventions and progressive changes are now in jeopardy. We can only hope that the strides made for women and the rights of others who are covered by these laws will sustain the backlash that confronts us.

One of the repercussions of the Third Wave of feminism was greater access to sport for girls and women, which has benefited us physically and psychologically. As middle-aged women we did not directly benefit from Title IX in high school or college, but we did gain some benefits from the groundswell of interest in, availability of, and "permission" to participate in physical activity. Around the time when Title IX became the law, feminists encouraged more flexible gender roles and urged all girls and women to take ownership of their bodies and to see themselves as more than sexual beings. More recently, messages about body image in the media have expanded to include the goal of fitness and the importance of a toned and healthy body.

However, gender stereotypes die hard(ly), and the culture still has a stranglehold on what women should look like. In the '60s Twiggy catapulted women into thinking that the androgynous look was the best. No longer was Marilyn Monroe, or women with contoured figures, the ideal. Our preoccupation with the perfect woman's body continues to prevail and influence who we are and our self-esteem. Body consciousness remains a volatile commodity, as most women have an unhealthy focus on appearance, a perspective reinforced by the media, commercialism, and a male-dominated economy.

The lives of women over 50 today are very different from the lives of our mothers and grandmothers. Modern technology has diminished the amount of physical labor required in many jobs and household chores, and the amount of discretionary time we have has increased. Baby boomers are living longer and healthier lives due to improvements in medicine and a greater knowledge of healthy lifestyles. Baby boomers reaped the benefits of the twentieth century's progress, and many of us have made a conscious effort to build physical activity into our schedules. Of course, there are many women who have physically demanding jobs (e.g., farming, domestic work, construction work). However, that work does not necessarily translate into better health. AARP (2002) reported that women who had physically demanding jobs were not necessarily healthier than those that did not.

More women are on the move. Trends in physical activity choices today include aerobics, Pilates, yoga, cycling, hiking, walking, team sports (e.g., field hockey), and master's level sporting and recreational events. The increased interest in sport and physical activity has been encouraged by the marketing of fitness: A greater variety of exercise gear is now made for women, including clothing and women's shoes and bicycles. Furthermore, there is an increased awareness and availability of healthy choices at the supermarket—foods with less salt and sugar, lower in fat, and with fewer carbohydrates make access to a healthy lifestyle easier to obtain. This being the case, why is the campaign for better fitness not reaching all women? Why is the body's need for regular physical activity not met by so many women over 50? What prevents women, especially middle-aged women, from becoming active in ways that increase our chances of aging that is guided by good health and fitness? Even though Title IX eluded us, middle-aged women certainly have opportunities their foremothers did not have, and we have the awareness that physical activity is essential to good health and a smart way to use our leisure time.

The purpose of this chapter is to address physical activity and its central role in women's pleasure in midlife. Whether physical activity involves a sport, exercise, or leisure activities, using our bodies is key to a healthy lifestyle. Integrating physical activity into daily living enhances the quality of life for women in a variety of ways. First I will define middle age and discuss how middle age affects women's bodies including the roles of health care and nutrition. Then I will provide an overview of physical activity and the results of the AARP study on physical activity for men and women over 50 and focus on women's midlife sport and leisure activities. A discussion of the effects of physical aging on the body and the importance of the duration and frequency of exercising will follow. Next I will discuss at-risk populations, the ramifications of physical inactivity, and the barriers to exercise. Ways to overcome exercise barriers will be addressed in terms of three niches that exercise fills: fun, competence, and confidence building. I will conclude with suggestions for future research, which is sorely needed.

What Is Middle Age?

Levinson (1996) referred to ages 50 to 55 as the Age 50 Transition, 55 to 60 as the Culmination of Middle Adulthood, and age 60 as the beginning of the Late Adult Transition. He described the Age 50 Transition as "an opportunity to reappraise the Entry Life Structure, to engage in some further exploration of self and world and to create a basis for the structure to be formed in the ensuing period" (p. 26), whereas 55 to 60 years of age is "...a vehicle for the realization of the era's majority aspiration and goals" (p. 26). Although Levinson did not address physical activity, sport, and exercise directly, these fit nicely into his notion of building in exercise as a cornerstone of one's quality of life.

Physical Changes in Middle Adulthood for Women

The physical changes that accompany middle adulthood for women, first and foremost, are the changes brought about by menopause—when a woman no longer has her menstrual period and her ability to reproduce ends. Although a colleague of mine recently announced the arrival of menopause with sadness and the loss of her child-bearing years, other women rejoice in the freedom from sanitary pads and tampons. Symptoms that accompany menopause vary from woman to woman. However, the diminished level of estrogen affects all women. Decreased muscle tone and a slower metabolism are features of menopause (MayoClinic.com, 2006; WebMD, 2006) that contribute to weight gain in middle-aged women. Consequently, middle-aged women are more at risk for becoming obese, and with obesity comes an increased risk of several chronic illnesses. Middle age is a time when chronic illnesses often emerge (Woods & Mitchell, 1997). These include heart disease, arthritis, hypertension, orthopedic problems, diabetes, asthma, chronic sinusitis, and bronchitis (National Center for Health Statistics, 1993).

Health Care and Nutrition Concerns

The disparity in access to good health care services has a trickle down effect on women's fitness. Mutschler and Alcon (1997) pointed out that there is a lack of quality health care for many women, especially older women and Women of Color and that the lack of adequate health care, along with the lack of emphasis on women's health concerns in research, jeopardizes those women's health. Poor health care can lead to chronic health problems that could have been avoided, and these health problems compromise women's quality of life and make it difficult for many to exercise regularly.

Nutrition is important to the health and quality of life of middle-aged women. If an individual has not had proper health care or nutrition, such exercise cannot have the optimal benefit. Virtually all products in the grocery store have labels to indicate their contents. There is more information in the media these days about the benefits of various nutrients and the portions necessary to maintain good nutrition. Yet, for many, old habits die hard, and modifications in the types of food eaten, as well as portion control, are a challenge. Fast and inexpensive food often translates into foods that are high in fat, sodium, sugar, and/or carbohydrates—the staples of the American diet. Fresh vegetables and fruits—mainstays of healthy eating—are perceived to be more expensive than the snack foods habits (e.g., chips, doughnuts, croissants, candy) that are common in American eating habits. In reality access especially to fresh fruit and vegetables at affordable prices is the real issue. Programs such as The Food Trust in Philadelphia (www.thefoodtrust.org) provide low-income neighborhoods with reasonably priced healthy foods in convenient locations, as well as nutrition education and demonstrate healthier ways to prepare food. Eating more healthfully is, for many, not only a conscious choice, but a concerted effort that requires modification in buying habits, food preparation, and taste preferences. AARP (2002) reported that 86% of women think that eating right is important to health. However, knowledge does not always translate into action.

Health care and nutrition complement physical activity as key components to fitness and maintaining a healthy weight in middle age. Most chronic illnesses (e.g., diabetes, hypertension, heart disease) of middle age are adversely affected by excess weight. Clearly, a healthy weight is central to a healthy life. Weil (2005) cautioned that "exercise by itself rarely corrects obesity unless it is accompanied by a change in eating habits, but it can prevent it, and ... regular aerobic exercise is absolutely necessary to maintain optimum health" (p. 181). Woods and Mitchell (1997) stated that "three of the most important risk factors for diseases that account for morbidity and mortality during the middle and older years are smoking, the quality of dietary intake, and sedentary lifestyle" (p. 74). Therefore, Levinson's suggested review of our lives and selves during middle age should include an assessment of eating habits and activity levels (Levinson, 1996).

Physical Activity, Exercise, and Physical Fitness

What exactly are we talking about when we say "physical activity"? The Surgeon General's Report (U.S. Department of Health and Human Services, 1996) made the following distinctions:

Physical activity: "Physical activity is defined as bodily movement produced by the contraction of skeletal muscle that increases energy expenditure above the basal level. Physical activity can be categorized in various ways, including type, intensity and purpose" (p. 20);

Exercise (or exercise training): "... exercise has been used to denote a subcategory of physical activity: physical activity that is planned, structured, repetitive and purposive in the sense that improvement and maintenance of one or more components of physical fitness is the objective" (Caspersen, Powell, & Christensen, 1985, as cited in U.S. Department of Health and Human Services, 1996, p. 20);

Physical fitness: "... the ability to carry out daily tasks with vigor and alertness, without undue fatigue, and with ample energy to enjoy leisure time pursuits and to meet unforeseen emergencies.... Health-related fitness includes cardiorespiratory fitness, muscular strength and endurance, body composition and flexibility" (p. 20);

Health: Bouchard, Shephard, Stephens, Sutton, and McPherson (1990, as cited in U.S. Department of Health and Human Services, 1996) stated that health is "... a human condition with physical, social and psychological dimensions, each characterized on a continuum with positive and negative poles. Positive health is associated with a capacity to enjoy life and to withstand challenges; it is not merely the absence of disease. Negative health is associated with morbidity and, in the extreme, with premature mortality" (p. 22).

Thus, good health, the ultimate goal, is contingent upon using our bodies in a manner that enhances our fitness. All middle-aged women must make a conscious effort to incorporate physical activity into their daily routines. Clearly, exercise is a factor in quality of life, for without physical fitness, we cannot continue to excel in the workplace, play with our grandchildren, or enjoy hobbies and other leisure pursuits, such as gardening and travel activities, that bring pleasure to the lives of so many midlife women.

Types of Exercisers

In May 2002, AARP conducted a survey on the exercise attitudes and behaviors of adults age 50 to 79. Two thousand men and women participated in a telephone interview of 15 to 20 min and responded to questions about their exercise habits. AARP (2002) identified six broad categories of types that describe why middle-aged and older adults exercise: socializers, matintainers, mind and body, the infirm, unmotivateds, and hectics. Women tended to be the following types: mind and body (exercise for fitness and the psychological benefits), unmotivated (tend not to exercise), the infirm (have health problems that compromise their ability to exercise), the hectics (no time), and the maintainers (exercise for health reasons). Only the socializer group was dominated by men (to have fun, to socialize, and to have a better sex life). Sixty-one percent of American women realize that exercise is important to good health yet they do not exercise (AARP, 2002). As one woman told me, "I don't get anything out of it."

The Effect of Physical Aging on the Body

Bone Strength and Osteoporosis

Musculoskeletal changes that occur with aging include osteoporosis and osteoarthritis and reduced muscle strength (Bassey et al., 2002). According to the

U.S. Department of Health and Human Services (1996), "...osteoarthritis is the leading cause of activity limitation among older persons" (p. 129). Women in Western societies are especially affected by these changes, which can lead to chronic illnesses and even death. Aging slows the process of bone cell growth, and thus the replacement of new bone cells for old ones lessens (Bassey et al., 2002). Although bone loss varies from woman to woman, the effects of menopause (e.g., the lower amounts of estrogen) exacerbate bone loss. Hormone replacement therapy (HRT) can curtail bone loss in postmenopausal women but many women are opposed to HRT for philosophical and political reasons, as well as the complications (e.g., cancer, increased risk of strokes) that may arise from it. Smaller, fair skinned women are especially vulnerable to osteoporosis and bone fractures with age (OB/GYN Reference Desk, 2006). Weight bearing exercises (e.g., resistance training, aerobics) are recommended as physical activity aids in managing the symptoms of osteoarthritis. Also increased calcium intake and pharmaceutical treatments such as Fosamax can help to build bone strength. Regarding osteoporosis, exercise decreases bone loss in postmenopausal women, although there is some debate about whether resistance or endurance is best (President's Council on Physical Fitness and Sports, 2006).

Joints and Osteoarthritis

According to Murray and Lopez (1990, as cited in Bassey et al., 2002, p. 151), "...osteoarthritis is the fourth most frequent cause of health problems in women worldwide." Osteoarthritis is the result of the loss of cartilage, which in turn causes pain, sensitivity, and swelling in the joints. Knees and wrists are especially vulnerable to osteoarthritis because they are two joints with repetitive movements (Cooper, 1994). Weil (2005) emphasized that repetition of the same activity can cause stress on specific body parts; the knees are particularly susceptible to overuse. You may wonder if exercise worsens the vulnerability of your joints. However, using your muscles and bones through exercise actually can aid in maintaining healthy joints. Stronger muscles around the knee can take some of the pressure off of the knee joint. It is under use of joints, inadequate nutrition, and excessive weight that can exacerbate problems. The key is to find exercises that do not cause damage to your joints (e.g., the elliptical machine). Although you may have to give up tennis, you can take up water aerobics or brisk walking. There is some truth in the adage "Use it or lose it."

Muscle Strength

Muscles not only help to stabilize bones and joints but they also aid in increasing the metabolism and burning calories (Weil, 2005). Aging shrinks the body's muscle mass by one-third to one-fifth, but this loss can be delayed by physical activity (Fiatarone et al., 1990, as cited in Bassey et al., 2002). In summary, all three factors—muscle strength, flexible joints, and bone density—are critical to healthy living, and all three are affected by aging. Healthy muscles, joints, and bones enhance both flexibility and balance. In turn, flexibility and balance aid in coordination. Actions such as standing and sitting, walking, getting dressed, leisure activities (e.g., gardening), sport, and exercise are all affected by an ability to be limber and balanced. Physical activity has a positive effect on our muscles, joints, bones, as well as our sense of balance and our flexibility. Flexible people are less likely to fall and, if they do fall, less likely to be injured. According to the AARP (2002) survey, 53% of women believe that flexibility is necessary. In addition, 46% of the women surveyed believe that strength training is important, and 36% believe that balance is very important. Both of the latter percentages were higher for women than for men. It is not surprising, then, that women gravitate toward yoga, Pilates, Tai Chi, and the use of exercise balls. Weil (2005) suggested that Hatha yoga, a more temperate form of yoga, is best for middle-aged and older adults.

In summary, as the U.S. Department of Health and Human Service (1996) stated, "Physical activity has numerous beneficial physiological effects. Most widely appreciated are its effect on the cardiovascular and musculoskeletal systems, but benefits on the functioning of metabolic, endocrine and immune systems are also considerable" (p. 7). The results of the AARP (2002) survey complement the findings of the U.S. Department of Health and Human Services, as they found that middle-aged and older adults report that their desire to exercise is fueled by "health benefits, improved appearance, personal satisfaction, and the opportunity to have fun and socialize ..." (p. 9). Physical activity helps to strengthen our skeleton. Physical activity, especially weight bearing physical activity, aids in sustaining bone mass, especially if the physical activity is done on a regular basis. Physical activity can aid in weight control, but it must be accompanied by good nutrition. The maintenance of an appropriate weight lessens stress on the body systems, including the skeleton and heart.

How Much Exercise Is Enough?

Physical activity need not be strenuous to achieve health benefits. The Surgeon General's Report (U.S. Department of Health and Human Services, 1996) stated that men and women of all ages benefit from even a moderate amount of daily physical activity. The Report recommended that exercise of at least moderate intensity for 30 min or more should be performed most, if not all, days of the week. A moderate amount of activity requires longer sessions (e.g., 30 min of brisk walking) whereas shorter sessions of more strenuous activities (e.g., 15 to 20 min of jogging) are also effective. AARP's survey indicated that 38% of the women surveyed thought that 30 min was an ample amount of time to exercise. However, it is important to remember that exercise must be at least 30 min in duration to begin burning fat. This will be discussed later.

Additional health benefits can be gained through greater amounts of physical activity. However, one must bear in mind that injury can accompany an increased level of physical activity. Middle-aged women who do not have a history of exercising vigorously should not begin with an unrealistically strenuous exercise program. Previously sedentary people who begin physical activity programs should start with short sessions (5 to 10 min) of physical activity and gradually build up to the desired level of activity (U.S. Department of Health and Human Services, 1996). Adults with chronic health conditions, such as heart disease, diabetes, or obesity, or who are at high risk for these conditions, should consult a physician before beginning a new program of physical activity. Men over age 40 and women over age 50 who plan to begin a new program of vigorous activity should consult a physician to be sure they do not have heart disease or other health problems.

At-Risk Populations

According to the U.S. Department of Health and Human Services (1996), "Physical inactivity is more prevalent among women than men, among Blacks and Hispanics than Whites, among older than younger adults, and among the less affluent than the more affluent" (p. 8). As there are more women and more Women of Color occupying low-income status in the United States, it is no surprise that class, race, and gender are intimate bedfellows (Hall, 1998). For example, using education as a measure of socioeconomic status, Grzywacz et al. (2004) found that people who are less educated report more severe stressors in their lives, which reinforces the notion that physical health, mental health, and stress are interconnected. The relationship between discretionary income, discretionary time, and safe environments contribute to low levels of exercise in communities of Color. Krause (2000) pointed out that there are a disproportionate number of women, especially Women of Color, who are poor. Concerns about access to health care may draw attention away from a focus on and an appreciation of physical activity as a preventive health measure. Socioeconomic status affects accessibility of services in heath and in health prevention, as well as accessibility of safe and convenient places to exercise (e.g., safe green spaces in the city), which, in turn, influence the desire to participate in physical activities.

Floyd et al. (1994) used the marginality and ethnicity hypotheses in their examination of leisure activity preferences (not participation) of Black and White women and men. The marginality hypothesis focuses on how socioeconomic status (i.e., limited time and money) affects leisure activity preferences, whereas the ethnicity hypothesis addresses the role of cultural norms in leisure activity preferences. Floyd and his associates found race differences between low income Blacks and Whites in leisure activity preferences, mainly among women, but not among middle income Black and White women. Thus, for middle class Black women, class supersedes race in preferred leisure activities. However, Blacks, regardless of class, rank exercise and socializing (e.g., parties; visiting friends and family; church, club, and voluntary activities) as preferred activities more than do Whites, who rank outdoor activities (e.g., bicycling, swimming) higher than Blacks do. Floyd et al. concluded that it was not culture or class that distinguished low income Black women, but it is the interaction of race and class that accounted for their dissimilar leisure activity preferences. They attributed this phenomenon to the discrimination that low income Black women face as Blacks, as poor, and as women. Their data are important to consider when we suggest exercise preferences with the race and socioeconomic status of the women in mind.

According to the 1991 National Health Interview Survey (U.S. Department of Health and Human Services, 2004), women, especially Blacks and Latinas, participate less than men do in strengthening activities, and their participation in strengthening activities declines with age. However, women do participate more in stretching activities than men do, and this remains relatively consistent until age 75. Again, education and income are also related to physical activity, as poorer and less educated adults tend to be less involved than more affluent and better educated adults 55 and older in all types of physical activity (Schoenborn et al., 2006).

The Ramifications of Physical Inactivity

Overall the absence of physical activity takes a toll on our bodies. More than 60% of U.S. adults do not engage in the recommended amount of activity, and approximately 25% of U.S. adults are not active at all (U.S. Department of Health and Human Services, 1996). Physical inactivity is more common among women than men, among African Americans and Hispanic Americans than European Americans, among older than younger adults, and among the less affluent than the more affluent. In addition, social support from family and friends has been consistently and positively related to regular physical activity. Although 36% of the women in AARP's survey indicated that they had exercised regularly for the past year or more, 30% stated that they did not engage in any regular physical activity. The highest percentage of women (39%) in AARP's survey indicated that they had exercised only occasionally throughout their lives.

Barriers to Exercise

Although many women over 50 know that they should exercise, their reasons for not exercising loom large and are roadblocks to following an exercise program. AARP's survey showed that the biggest barrier is lack of time, followed by fatigue, and health problems (AARP, 2002). The health problems most commonly referenced were arthritis, chronic pain, injury, physical disabilities, and heart problems. In addition, lack of desire, inconvenient locations, safety concerns, and the lack of an exercise history prevent middle-aged women from exercising. AARP also found that safety, low-cost facilities, and having an exercise companion are important precursors to regular exercise. Some middle-aged women prefer to take classes, especially weight lifting, strength training, and aerobics. One hypothesis for the success of classes is that they are structured and provide instruction, which women may find appealing, and this is especially so for middle-aged women who are self-conscious because of their body image, unfamiliar with exercise equipment, or inexperienced in workout routines. For example, *Curves* is a women only facility, and many women like it because they prefer to avoid the "meat market" atmosphere associated with coed gyms. However, for the most part, it seems that middle-aged women do not see exercise and physical activity as a priority.

Midlife is a busy time for women's careers and family responsibilities. It is a time during which many women begin caretaking of their parents or in-laws. Community involvement may also be time consuming for many women. Commuting to and from work is another commitment that takes away from personal time. Given these responsibilities, building in an exercise program, for many women, is less attractive than other priorities, especially if they have never had the opportunity to build in an exercise program in the past.

Why Begin? Why Persist?

Women are more likely than men to begin to exercise for weight loss (30% versus 24%, respectively); other common motivations are staying fit and for purposes of their health (AARP, 2002). I often speak with middle-aged women regarding exercise, and the vast majority of them, especially Black women, say that they exercise because of their health, either as a preventive measure or as a means to slow down the progression of a chronic illness. These same women say that it is the consequences of the exercise that maintains their physical activity. "I feel so good afterwards, that's why I do it, and it's good for me," commented one 58-year-old woman. "I didn't exercise before but I want to be flexible as I age. I work for the phone company and spend plenty of time on a ladder, but water aerobics helps me to stay flexible." To paraphrase another 50+ woman, "Since I began Aikido, I can knock down a man. That makes me feel great!"

The Pleasures of Exercising

There are many women who enjoy exercise and physical activity. The sense of competence that grows from exercising is rewarding, whether it is an increase in endurance, greater mastery and skill in the execution of a sport, the pleasure in using the body in a physical activity, the "alone time" that some exercise offers, or the feeling of camaraderie that emerges from team sports and leisure activities. The process of gaining skills and confidence in a sport or an exercise routine is exciting and reinforces the desire to exercise more. Many women who have careers where the beginning and end of a project spans weeks or months enjoy exercise sessions because they are finite and gratifying because you can complete what you set out to do. Although the overall cost–benefit may take time (e.g., weight loss, body toning), the sense of completion is, itself, rewarding. One of my colleagues loves to garden, and the enjoyment she receives from growing flowers is important to her mental health and sense of satisfaction. Another woman told me that she likes to swim because it is the only time that someone is not calling her name ("Mom," "Honey," "Professor," etc.); swimming provides her with a time to think and to process. Another middle-aged women I know loves field hockey and the satisfaction she receives from being part of a group.

As Levinson (1996) suggested, middle age is a time for both reflecting and doing; we create a stage for our personal growth, which often includes a new or renewed commitment to a spiritual path as well as an assessment of our physical well-being.

Not only does exercise prevent disease, but it also improves one's quality of life (U.S. Department of Health and Human Services, 1996). Physical exercise helps with sleep problems (Flora, 2003), stress, and depression (Berger et al., 2002). Clearly an overall sense of well-being is a common byproduct of physical activity, as are feelings of competence (Berger et al., 2002). Exercise actually gives us more energy, and the fatigue that accompanies vigorous workouts generates feelings of satisfaction and accomplishment. As a psychotherapist and sport psychologist, I regularly recommend the benefits of exercise to my sedentary clients.

Types of Physical Activity

Both aerobic and anaerobic exercises are important to physical fitness. Aerobic exercise carries oxygen to the working muscles. Aerobic activity is focused on cardiovascular conditioning, and it is important to maintaining the heart and blood flow (Berger et al., 2002; Weil, 2005). Examples of aerobic or cardiovascular fitness activities include walking up the stairs, swimming, cardio kickboxing, step classes, and brisk walking. Low impact aerobic activities include brisk walking, stationary cycling, bicycling, jogging, running, and swimming (Weil, 2005). The AARP (2002) survey showed that brisk walking, cycling, vacuuming, and gardening for at least 20 min were the preferred physical activities of older women. AARP also found that men were more likely to participate in a sport, whereas women were more likely to identify their physical activity in terms of household chores. Most women (73%) said that they exercised in the home.

Anaerobic exercise complements aerobic or cardiovascular fitness by stressing systems that strengthen muscles. Anaerobic exercises use muscles for a short period of time (e.g., weight lifting), but do not transport oxygen to the working muscles. The burning of fat is what most exercisers are interested in doing. According to Health Education Associates (2006), glycogen, a sugar stored in the muscle tissues, is activated and used as fuel for the first 3 min of exercise. When glycogen is burned during intense exercising, the burn that you feel in your muscles is the lactic acid that created by the burning of glycogen. "Once these stores of glycogen are used up, which usually occurs after about 20 min, the body will start burning its fat stores to produce blood sugar and ultimately glycogen. The longer you exercise the more fat burned. Body fat produces energy for exercising" (Health Education Associates, 2006). Resistance training can increase muscle strength and density, which, in turn, burns fat, and people burn more calories with muscles than with fat (MayoClinic.com, 2006). The U.S. Department of Health and Human Services (1996) has recommended that strength training should be added to an aerobic routine for musculoskeletal health 2 days each week.

Selection of a Physical Activity

Middle-aged women should select a physical activity that they will enjoy and one that they are able to do. Running is frequently thought of as "the" preferred physical activity. However, if a woman is not a runner, there is no need to begin to run or jog, as there are many other options. Running is hard on the joints; brisk walking is, by far, a preferred aerobic activity of middle-aged women and one that is supported by the Surgeon General. Swimming, biking, elliptical machines, ergometers, and treadmills are other options that contribute to a stronger heart, better blood circulation, lower blood pressure, and speed up the slower metabolism that accompanies middle age. Aerobic and step classes, as previously mentioned, are also good alternatives. The goal should be to keep the heart rate within the target heart rate (THR). The simplest way for women to find out their THR is to begin by calculating their maximum heart rate (MHR). This is done by subtracting one's age from 226. Next, determine the resting heart rate (RHR), and subtract this number from the previous number. Last, multiply this number (MHR minus RHR) by .60 and .85 to determine your THR range.

> For example:
> Age: 55
> 226
> $\underline{-55}$
> $171 \times .60 = 103$
> $171 \times .85 = 145$
> THR $= 103$–145 heartbeats/min.

We have achieved a certain amount of success if we can talk while participating in the activity (swimming is an exception). Another sign of success is the lowering of the recovery rate after exercise. The better shape people are in, the quicker their heart rate returns to their normal number of beats per minute after strenuous activity.

Sports and Master Level Athletes

Just because women get older does not mean that they lose their competitive nature in sport. Master level athletes are older people who compete within their age range for prizes or recognition in their event. Master's level events also apply to sports before the age of 50 (e.g., runners in their 30s), but the intent is to have similar aged athletes in competition with each other. For example, Billie Jean King would compete in events for women over 50, and as of October 18, 2006, Martina Navratilova will have received her AARP card. There are a growing number of middle-aged women who are master's level athletes in sports including rowing (Nordon, 2003), swimming, soccer, and running (Jokl et al., 2004). Anywhere there's a sport, we are likely to find a middle-aged (or older) women participating! For the most part, master's women athletes participated in sports when they were younger, but many, who are looking for exercise and a social network of women, train and enter master's level activities for the challenge and the sense of gratification that comes with a competitive atmosphere. This select group of women is continuing to grow and will undoubtedly increase as post-Title IX women become card-carrying members of AARP.

Quality of Life and Conclusion

It is interesting that data on adults and physical activity were not collected until the 1980s (U.S. Department of Health and Human Services, 1996). In my review of the literature on women in midlife, there were surprisingly articles specific to this age group on exercise and leisure activities. I was surprised and not certain why there is this void. Sherry Willis stated that "some researchers say middle age is really dull because nothing happens" and changes in later adulthood are more interesting to researchers as the changes are more significant (Clay, 2003, p. 36). Midlife women are caught between an emphasis on the 40s and the "retirement age" of 65. Clearly future research must be conducted that targets women in midlife. AARP's study is a beginning. With the increasing lifespan of women, there is an even greater need to focus on health issues and prevention for many reasons, including the rising cost of health care, but most important is the quality of life as we age. We need to examine subpopulations of midlife women including the commonalities and differences in exercise and physical activities related to socioeconomic status, race, ethnicity, disability, and sexual orientation. Future research should also include a more detailed approach to understanding exercise adherence. For example, what makes women begin to exercise again after they stopped? We have an idea why women stop, but the stop and start patterns of women in their 50s would be interesting to explore. Research should include an investigation of why certain exercise, leisure activities, or sports activities are selected, whether women's choices of exercise change over time (and why), and how prior exercise history before age 50 influences their decisions.

What we do know is clear. The overall message of the research on adults in midlife is simple: Keep moving! Living through middle age is not just about biding time. It's about living! Midlife is a time when women and men begin to reflect and become aware that the time ahead of them is shorter than the time that they have lived so far. As such, personal inventories and lifestyles are often assessed, and modifications are made to maintain a good quality of life. Exercise can enhance our quality of life in a variety of ways including physical health, energy level, a better mood, stress management, and skills building (Berger et al., 2002). We need to encourage young women to begin an exercise routine for self care and remind them that exercise can become a family activity (e.g., biking, walking, boating, gardening together). Or it can be an "alone time"—a time to get in touch with ourselves in a healthful and pleasurable way. However, it is never too late for people who have not been physically active to begin. Middle-aged women are usually well established in their employment and community activities. For middle-aged women, the exercise mantra should be "Do it for yourself." It is time to enjoy the fruits of our labor. Beginning with a physical checkup is a good idea for middle-aged and older women and for any woman who has not exercised previously (U.S. Department of Health and Human Services, 1996). Regardless of age, people should begin slowly and build up their endurance by doing a limited amount of physical activity for a short duration. They should find a physical activity that they might enjoy and one that they are willing to make part of their lifestyle. The key is to make physical activity as important as other necessities in life such as sleeping and eating. If people "fall off the wagon" and hit periods of inactivity, they should simply begin again. Life is full of stops and starts, and exercise programs are no exception. Remember that the benefits of physical activity diminish after 2 weeks, and if physical activity is stopped for 2 to 8 months, the cost benefit of previous efforts is erased (U.S. Department of Health and Human Services, 1996). Keeping up an exercise program is easier for most women if they find a friend, who can act as a motivator and as someone to whom they are accountable. Exercising with a friend makes it more enjoyable for most women.

Gender, race, age, social class, and health status all affect the physical activity of middle-aged women. With middle age, gravity is making itself known. Wrinkles are here to stay. Many of us have lost and found the same pounds over and over again. We're on our nth gym membership. However, when we hit 50 we don't care as much about small things and, simultaneously, we realize the importance of our own needs and priorities. I'm reminded of Towanda, the alter ego of Evelyn Couch (played by Kathy Bates), in the film *Fried Green Tomatoes,* who said: "I'm too old to be young and too young to be old." It is unfortunate that many of us have not made exercise a priority. Motivation is a major factor that needs to be addressed. However, in sport, like the rest of life, nothing is as simple as it appears. Sometimes life and exercise are most aptly reflected in the Nike slogan "Just Do It." We do not have to process completing our exercise for the day; we just need to do it. Some days are harder than others, but, in the long run, making exercise part of daily life is worthwhile. I hope that, with more role models, greater access to facilities, and continued media visibility about the importance of exercise, changes will continue to be made. We are the generation that worked to ensure that girls have the same rights as boys to sport and physical activities. We saw the manufacture and marketing of sporting goods and clothing that was specific to women's bodies so that women no longer had to use men's hand-me-downs. Middle age is a time when many women begin to explore what is out there in the world for them—what we missed and what we want to do. It is a time to get reacquainted with our playfulness. Yes, physical activity is self-care, but it is also fun. And we deserve it.

References

American Association of Retired People (AARP). (2002). *Exercise Attitudes and Behaviors: A Survey of Adults Age 50–79.* Washington, DC: AARP.

Bassey, J., Sayer, A.A., and Cooper C. (2002). A life course approach to musculoskeletal aging: Muscle strength, osteoporosis, and osteoarthritis. In D. Kuh and R. Hardy (Eds.), *A Life Course Approach to Women's Health* (pp. 141–160). New York: Oxford University Press.

Berger, B., Pargman, D., and Weinberg, R.S. (2002). *Foundations of Exercise Psychology.* Morgantown, VA: Fitness Information Technology, Inc.

Cooper, D. (1994). Osteoarthritis epidemiology. In J.H. Klippel and P.A. Dieppe (Eds.), *Rheumatology* (pp. 731–734). St. Louis, MO: Mosby.

Clay, R.A. (2003, April). Researchers replace midlife myths with facts: Job changes and stress management can positively affect midlife health. *APA Monitor*, pp. 34, 36.

Flora, C. (2003, November). Exercise helps sleep in menopause. *Psychology Today*, p. 25.

Floyd, M.F., Shinew, K.J., McGuire, F.A., and Noe, F.P. (1994). Race, class, and leisure activity preferences: Marginality and ethnicity revisited. *Journal of Leisure Research, 26*, 158–173.

Grzywacz, J.G., Almeida, D.M. Neupert, S.D., and Ettner, S.L. (2004). Socioeconomic status and health: A micro-level analysis of exposure and vulnerability to daily stressors. *Journal of Health and Social Behavior, 45*, 1–16.

Hall, R.L. (1998). Softly strong: African American women's use of exercise in therapy. *Psychotherapy Patient, 10*(3/4), 81–100.

Health Education Associates. [retrieved March 5, 2006]. *Aerobic Versus Anaerobic Exercise*. http://www.well-net.com/cardiov/aerex1.html).

Jokl, P., Sethi, P.M., and Cooper, A.J. (2004). Master's performance in the New York City Marathon. *British Journal of Sports Medicine, 38*, 408–412.

Krause, M. (2000). Are we really entering a new era of aging? In K.W. Schaie and J. Hendricks (Eds.), *The Evolution of the Aging Self: The Societal Impact on the Aging Process* (pp. 307–318). New York: Springer.

Levinson, D.J. (1996). *The Seasons of a Woman's Life*. New York: Knopf.

Nordon, K. (2003, May 7). Hitting their stride. *Christian Science Monitor*. http://www.csmonitor.com/atcsmonitor/specials/women/sports/sports050703.html.

MayoClinic.com. (retrieved April 12, 2006). *Menopause and Weight Gain: Reverse Middle Aged Spread*. http://www.mayhoclinic.com/health/menopause-weight-gain/HQ01076.

Mutschler, P.H., and Alcon, A. (1997). Health concerns in midlife and older women: Improving the quality of women's live as they age [Electronic Version]. *National Council of Jewish Women Journal, 20*, 22–26.

National Center for Health Statistics. (1993). Advance report of final mortality statistics, 1991. *Monthly Vital Statistics Report, 42*(2). Hyattsville, MD: Author.

OB/GYN Reference Desk. (retrieved April 13, 2006). *Menopause and Midlife Health for Women*. http://www.umanitoba.ca/womens_health/meno5.htm.

President's Council on Physical Fitness and Sports (retrieved February 26, 2006). *Fitness fundamentals*. [http://www.hoptechno.com/book11.htm].

Schoenborn, C.A., Vickerie, J.L., and Powell-Griner, E. (2006, April 11). Health characteristics of adults 55 years of age Andover: United States, 2000–2003. *Advance Data from Vital and Health Statistics, 370*. http://www.cdc.gov/nchs/data/ad/ad370.pdf.

Schultz, S. (1999, November 8). Why we're fat. *U.S. News & World Report*, pp. 82–85.

The Food Trust. (2006, April 19). *The Next Decade: Building Strong Communities Through Healthy Food*. http://www.thefoodtrust.org/catalog/download.php?product_id=69.

U.S. Department of Health and Human Services Center for Disease Control and Prevention. (2004). *1991 National Health Interview Survey*. Hyattsville, MD: National Center for Health Statistics. http://www.cdc.gov/nchs/products/elec_prods/subject/nhis.htm

U.S. Department of Health and Human Services. (1991). *Healthy People 2000: National Health Promotion and Disease Prevention Objectives—Full Report with Commentary*. Washington, DC: U.S. Department of Health and Human Services.

U.S. Department of Health and Human Services. (1996). *Physical Activity and Health: A Report of the Surgeon General*. Washington, DC: U.S. Department of Health and Human Services.

WebMD Medical Reference in collaboration with the Cleveland Clinic. (2006, February 13). *Menopause Basics.* http//www.webmd.com/content/article/51/40624.htm.

Weil, A. (2005). *Healthy Aging.* New York: Knopf.

Woods, N.F., and Mitchell, E.S. (1997). Preventive health issues: The perimenopausal to mature years (45–64). In K.M. Allen and J.M. Phillips (Eds.), *Women's Health across the Lifespan: A Comprehensive Perspective* (pp. 72–89). Philadelphia: Lippincott.

5
The Well-being and Quality of Life of Women Over 50: A Gendered-Age Perspective

Varda Muhlbauer

In recent decades renewed attention has been given to the notion of middle age and particularly to women in this age group. Many of us think that this is a welcome development. These women (popularly referred to as "baby boomers") have capitalized on the major sociocultural changes and transformed meanings and behavioral codes traditionally attached to this age group. In numerous interviews, in both academic and popular media, the dominant sentiment voiced by middle-aged women is of overall satisfaction, to the effect that "the puzzle [life issues] straightens out...there is a greater sense of confidence in relations and overall a greater sense of authenticity...now it is totally me." The discussion becomes complicated, however, when issues related to body image and, particularly, sex appeal are raised. Statements such as "I feel invisible...I don't attract men" can be heard. It is as though there has been a trade-off: a sense of greater self-assertion in return for vulnerability vis-à-vis desirability and romance. Therefore, issues related to well-being and the quality of life of women in this age group cannot be easily measured. In this chapter I will discuss changes in gendered-age roles of women in this age group and the fragmented structure of well-being that results.

It is clear that any debate concerning the well-being of women in midlife involves both personal and social issues. To a large extent, well-being is the outcome of an ongoing interchange between sociocultural influences and human agencies (Blaikie, 1999). In this process, women proactively construct their personal experiences within conceptual and normative boundaries delineated by powerful sociocultural factors. This view is supported by the social construction perspective advocated by such diverse disciplines as cultural anthropology, social gerontology, social psychology, sociology, and feminist studies (Gergen, 1985; Gergen, 1990; Kaufman, 1986). One of the basic tenets of social construction is that social constructs are not the direct and inevitable outcome of forces of nature (a point of view often termed "essentialist" and indicative of a biological bias driven by political and cultural interests). They are, rather, "social artifacts, products of historically situated interchanges among people" (Gergen, 1985, p. 267). Thus, the major organizing principles of psychosocial experience and well-being, among them gender and age, have attracted considerable theoretical interest, and political attention, and in some contexts are even viewed as sensitive issues.

Feminist researchers and theorists have pioneered studies of the ways in which the dominant culture attaches gendered meanings to a large variety of psychosocial experiences, thereby influencing every aspect of women's lives. These culturally constructed meanings are shaped into gender roles that appear to be so basic to people's lives that it requires a conscious effort to focus on how they have been produced (Lorber, 1994). The construction and maintenance of gender roles and a gendered hierarchy, and the psychosocial problems associated with them, are among the leading issues that have been investigated (Collins, 1998). The similarities discovered among women (e.g., domains of power and powerlessness), despite individual differences, reveal that common cultural notions of gender play an important role in establishing well-being and expectations regarding possible life styles. Nonetheless, gender is basically a flexible social category subject to constantly evolving cultural meanings and shifts in power structures. Consequently, even a constructed consensus regarding gendered meanings does not exclude the existence of an ongoing process of alteration and modification (whether gradual and subversive or swift and overt), either on a personal or an institutional level.

Age is an equally important core socio-cultural construct, which is currently attracting unprecedented attention similar to the earlier interest in gender. Although age is undoubtedly linked to demographic, social, and cultural changes, the constructionist orientation again stresses the interdependence of aging and sociocultural changes, as each can transform the other. Frequent references are made to the need to redefine the borderlines between age groups and the growing salience of middle age (Neugarten & Neugarten, 1996). New terms, such as "young-old," are being coined to adapt to a changing reality. Thus, age is as subject to changes in perception as is gender, because age, too, is dependent upon social and cultural developments and adjustments in power structures (Blaikie, 1999).

The major cultural shifts of the last four decades are clearly reflected in revised gendered-age roles. These changes are particularly pronounced for women in midlife (Friedman, 1996). Given the assumption that self-definition and lifestyle options are realigned over time as social circumstances change (Gergen, 1985), the alteration in gendered-age roles is of considerable importance for the well-being of women at midlife. I will attempt here to demonstrate the link between the new sociocultural meanings of gendered-age roles and well-being that have resulted from societal shifts in the gendered-age balance of power. Power, a complicated construct in itself, not only enhances people's self-esteem and self-confidence, rather, it "increases the boundaries of what is achievable" (Mosedale, 2005, p. 250). It is, therefore, assumed that power roles (particularly accessible to privileged members of this group) constitute an important feature of the requisite repertoire of behaviors for positive functioning and overall well-being. Consequently, the current process of blurring and diversifying age and gender roles allows for greater access to power structures and has, therefore, a positive impact on the psychological well-being of women over 50.

Although the modern emphasis on the "new" identities of middle-aged women is intended to celebrate this life stage, several constraints remain intact. These constraints are particularly conspicuous in contemporary sexualized societies (Arber et al., 2003). To a large extent, the common conceptions of the sexual attractiveness of women over 50 are still unchallenged, and continue to be seen through a man's perspective. Powell and Moores (2001) stated that this tendency is indicative of the pressure on women to comply with cultural standards of desirability and the degree of male domination in society. In addition, patterns of intimate relationships and partnerships are still negatively affected by the gendered-age role of women over 50. This is especially worrisome from the perspective of well-being, as the need for intimate relations does not change fundamentally through the life course, and such relationships are associated with sustained self-esteem and self-identity (Davidson & Fennell, 2002).

The popular media (e.g., television, the Internet, advertisements, newspapers, films) provide abundant illustrations of the fragmented shift in the perception of women over 50. Indeed, the connection between media representations and sociocultural constructs of gender and age cannot be overstated, so that documenting them is likely to enhance our understanding. With this in mind, Lauzen and Dozier (2005) analyzed the 100 top-grossing American films of 2002, and found evidence of a lingering double standard for aging women. They reported that female characters are, for the most part, kept frozen forever in their 20s and 30s. There are, however, a number of more innovative and daring trends that seem to incorporate a fresher approach in which gendered-age traditionalism is losing ground. The popular media therefore reflect the disjointed changes in the perception of gendered-age roles, particularly those of women aged 50 and over.

The Incomplete Shift in the Traditional Perception of the Feminine Gender Role

For many years, women over 50 figured in public and academic discourse largely in the context of traditional ideologies, which emphasized their reproductive and mothering functions. The almost exclusive focus on women as biological beings was borne out by an overview of textbooks and other professional literature (Gergen, 1990). The biological bias in accounts of women's adult development is linked to the normative structure of power. Powell and Moores (2001) claimed that dominant power conventions operate to connect women's status to their role in reproduction and to their youthfulness of appearance. Consequently, the cessation of reproductive capacities and the children's eventual departure from the home were almost exclusively viewed in terms of aging and loss. Similarly, the gradual loss of youthful appearance that occurs naturally in the course of life was bound with social devaluation and marginalization. The emphasis on disengagement from socially valued roles adversely affected the health and subjective sense of well-being of women over 50.

It is interesting to note that, although the complex of interconnections between cultural representations, central gender roles, self-concept, self-esteem, and well-being was at the core of feminist writings almost from the start, the marked impact it had on women over 50 was largely neglected. Even in the late1970s, Barnett and Baruch (1978) held that relatively little was known about the middle years and "particularly in respect to women, theoretical work is in its infancy, and empirical findings tend to be scattered and non-cumulative" (p. 187). They also drew attention to underlying biological assumptions in certain studies of women in midlife that exaggerate the importance of the reproductive role, the menopause, and the "empty nest," and they pointed to conflicting findings regarding the meanings that women attach to those events.

An iconoclastic approach to women in midlife was slow to come. When it did, however, the transition from concerns about the prevalence of depression among middle-aged women (Bart, 1971) to a view of middle age as the "prime of life" (Mitchell & Helson, 1990) was nothing less than revolutionary in nature. Mitchell and Helson described the early 50s as a junction between enhanced personal resources and a freer lifestyle made possible by the departure of grown children. They referred to this period as "an androgynous time of good health combined with autonomy and relational security" (p. 451). Burns and Leonard (2005) reported that women's perception of gain (in terms of satisfaction with life and stress relief) continues into the mid-60s and that the gains are related in part to role change and the passage of time. Additional studies (Helson & Moane, 1987; Helson & Wink, 1992) also contributed to a new interpretation of the period following menopause and the diminishing role of mothering. In these studies women in their 50s were found to be self-confident, secure, and better adjusted in their relationships.

The association between disengagement from traditional gender roles and cumulative personal resources on the one hand, and the quality of life in middle age on the other hand, is in sharp contrast to previous perceptions of this development in a woman's life. Obviously, the implications for the subjective well-being and lifestyle opportunities of women over 50 are enormous. Women today often welcome the cessation of menstruation, and they see new options available to them when their children leave home. In retrospect, this transformation can be attributed to a powerful blend of societal and conceptual changes, which have resulted from partial shifts in the balance of power structures, most particularly a greater diversity of gender and age roles and the widespread acceptance of a contextualized approach to gendered-age identities (Denmark, 1994; Ryff, 1987).

The reshaping of the quality of life patterns of many women is abundantly clear, and it helps women to confront serious issues in the realm of power and self-support. According to Helson (1997), whose findings were based on both self-descriptions and observers' ratings, women's competence increased significantly between the ages of 30 and 60. Stewart and Ostrove (1998) also referred to the development of a more effective instrumental personality in middle age.

Nonetheless, certain key concerns are still being largely ignored. These include the issues of body image, sex appeal, sexual relations, and romantic attachments. Although the literature on the institutional and personal power of women in their 50s (especially socially privileged women) explains their greater overall sense of well-being, it often describes them as though they were asexual and devoid of sexual needs. The mainstream media reinforce this image. Wolf (1998) claimed that, although women have more money, power, and recognition than ever before, they are worse off in terms of the way they feel about themselves physically. She has written that the cults of weight and age feed the terror of aging. In addition, the cultural construct of female sexuality still holds women to more restrictive standards than those for men (Peach, 1998). This sexist double-standard is quite conspicuous in middle age, when men are encouraged to be sexually active, often with much younger partners, whereas women are considered past the acceptable age for sexual activity. Wolf contended that this double-standard amounts to a counter-offensive against women.

A Twofold View of the Well-being of Women in Their 50s

Evidently, there is more than one way to view the issue of the quality of life and well-being of women over 50: the expansive view, wherein women enjoy a heightened consciousness of self, relative security, confidence, and a sense of growth and opportunity; and the contractive view, wherein they experience increased vulnerability and loss of confidence, mainly as a result of a sense of diminished physical and sexual attractiveness and inadequate intimate relationships. In one study, for example, Rossi (2004) found that loss of attractiveness was a source of worry for two-thirds of the interviewees in this age group, which indicates that the social and psychological significance of the menopausal transition lies in the experience of aging rather than in the loss of fertility. Indeed, any review (e.g., Peach, 1998; Strinati, 1995) of the cultural representations of women over 50 in contemporary popular culture reveals a heated debate with respect to the expansive versus contractive views of middle-aged women. The question, therefore, is how to reconcile these two contrasting notions of well-being.

One mark of health and psychological well-being is the capacity to integrate and successfully negotiate diverse needs. Ryff and Singer (1998) were critical of the tendency to "construe human health as exclusively about the mind or the body," and they called for a change in the direction of "an integrated and positive spiral of mind and body" (p. 1). However, the fragmented and divisive paradigm reflected in the expansive–contractive view of the well-being of women in midlife does not accommodate such integration. The access to personal power and real life achievements, often in competitive positions, does not relieve the stress and anxiety related to physical attraction, nor does it affect the likelihood of romantic attachments and sexual activity. Thus, only the needs associated with the expansive view are satisfied. The unattended needs may evoke negative thoughts and feelings and adversely affect the sense of well-being. It is reasonable to expect that the split (i.e., the rise and fall in cognition and affect) is replicated in women's real life experiences. This split complicates the attempt to arrive at a decisive and unidimensional evaluation of the well-being of women over 50.

The Expansive View

Well-being and Gender Roles

The meaning of well-being is typically multidimensional (Ryff & Keyes, 1995), elusive, controversial (Schmuck & Sheldon, 2001), and relative (Ryff, 1991), that is, individuals tend to see themselves as either getting better or worse over time. However, most theorists recognize the importance of two major aspects. The first is some combination of overall life satisfaction, positive affect, relative lack of negative affect (Cheng, 2004), and happiness (Ryff & Keyes, 1995; Schmutte & Ryff, 1997). The second is overall and positive functioning that is indicative of growth, self-sufficiency, autonomy, and a sense of mastery (Keyes et al., 2002). The concepts of mastery, autonomy, and self-efficacy associated with the positive functioning aspect of well-being easily resonate with what we know as the traditional masculine sociocultural construct. In this respect, not much has changed since the classic findings reported in the late '60s and '70s by Rosenkrantz et al. (1968) and by Broverman et al. (1970), who established the differential social desirability of the masculine and feminine gender roles and their relation to clinical judgments of mental health.

Gender roles continue to be a reference point for the analysis of well-being in more recent studies. However, the emphasis has now shifted to androgyny, that is, a balanced identity that combines stereotypically masculine and feminine personality characteristics (e.g., Helgeson, 1994; Helson & Picano, 1990; Woodhill & Samuels, 2003) and to the relationship between multiple social roles (which are usually indicative of greater gendered balance) and well-being (e.g., Pietromonaco et al., 1986; Thoits, 1983). Overall, it can be said that the expansive view of the well-being of women in their 50s relates to the acquisition of a more balanced composition of gendered characteristics and gendered roles.

Gender Role, Life Course, and Well-being

Developmental psychologists interested in changes across the life course have long argued that the tasks of early adulthood tend to polarize values and behaviors related to gender roles. This rigid gender role regime, often restrictive in nature, becomes more flexible in midlife, especially after the children leave home. Gutmann (1975) claimed that the conventionally distinctive gender role structure is a basic requirement of parenthood. This requirement ends when the children are grown and do not need the supportive behaviors associated with the early pattern of parenthood. The completion of tasks associated with one stage in the life course clears the way for renewal and the emergence of a different set of values and behaviors. Thus, in midlife, women tend to move in the direction of the masculine pole (i.e., toward increased instrumentality and assertiveness), and the aggressive inclinations that were suppressed in early adulthood are allowed to emerge (Neugarten & Gutmann, 1968). Similar arguments have been advanced by Livson (1976, 1981), who contended that shifting gender role expectations in middle age enable many women to grow and expand their psychological horizons: "Traditional sex roles, if taken for granted in early adulthood, may change or demand redefinition... Women who organized their identities around mothering may now be motivated to find new roles and sources of satisfaction" (Livson, 1981, p. 196). Thus, from a developmental perspective, for women the significance of the period following the intensively demanding parental years is related to a reshuffling of gender roles in ways that allow for more flexibility and greater acceptance of parts of themselves conventionally associated with the masculine gender role.

It goes without saying, however, that changes in gender identity and role expectations are not the same in all generations (Parker & Aldwin, 1997; Stewart & Healy, 1989) or social contexts. Midlife personality development and its implications for well-being must therefore be considered from a much broader sociocultural perspective. Although the links between the developmental processes (particularly changes related to life-course stage and role occupancy) and the larger sociocultural context (cohort and period effects) are far from simple, they can enhance our understanding of issues that pertain to the well-being and quality of life of women in their 50s.

Gender Role Identity, Social and Historical Developments, and Well-being

The expansive view of the well-being of women over 50 can be comprehended more easily if we take into account the huge impact of the feminist movement. Women now in their 50s were adolescents or young adults when the second wave of the feminist movement burst onto the scene, attracting immense interest and involvement across different age groups. The relevance of the feminist movement is particularly marked in respect to the shaping of the gender identity of this age group.

Among the movement's major goals was the reconstruction of women's roles on an expansive platform that would allow women to redefine relations, both at home and in the workplace, on the basis of equality. Stewart and Healy (1989) contended that the women who experienced the feminist movement while still in transition to adulthood (as did those in their 50s today) were deeply impressed by it, and incorporated its views in ways that have stayed with them for life. Indeed, they argued that any cohort-defining event of the caliber of the feminist movement tends to ascribe special prominence to evolving cohort norms, thus adding extra power to its initial molding effect.

As noted above, among the consequences of the social change brought about by the women's movement was a shift in society's views of appropriate roles for women. Welsh and Stewart (1995) maintained that the choices made by many women reflected a shift away from the role choices and experiences of their mothers and toward those of their fathers. Thus, the cohort of women now over 50 enjoyed the freedom to select adult roles while still in transition to adulthood (which is also the stage in which occupational identity is consolidated), and their choices bore a greater resemblance to men's roles than ever before.

The growing repertoire of diversified gender roles available to women who made their transition to adulthood in the 1960s is especially meaningful when viewed from the perspective of identity theory. Thoits (2003) argued that "we accept our positions and roles as identities [i.e., 'role identities']" (p. 179). Identities, in turn, have important mental health implications because they affect the ways that individuals think and feel about themselves and others. Consequently, the extensive selection of gender roles made available to women influenced the opportunities they had for role-identity acquisition and accumulation which, eventually, engendered resources for their well-being. The accumulation of role-identities enabled women to expand their capabilities, interests, and goals and to build up institutional and personal resources, often while retaining traditional responsibilities. As a result, women who have recently entered midlife have also experienced the labor market in a different way than previous generations.

Sexual Identity, Social–Historical Development, and Well-being

The 1960s saw not only the emergence of the feminist movement, but also the sexual revolution. Although the latter did not succeed in eliminating the sexual double standard (Peach, 1998), it had a strong impact on women's attitudes and behaviors. Ehrenreich et al. (1986) reported that it was women, not men, who changed fundamentally as a result of the sexual revolution, a finding confirmed by Baumeister's (2000) extensive review of relevant studies. The change is also evident when this generation is compared to older women who came of age before the sexual revolution (Laumann et al., 1994).

Nonetheless, the gains of the sexual revolution and later developments did not extend to older people in general or to older women in particular. Long-standing stereotypes continue to place middle-aged, and certainly elderly, women outside the sexualized world (Hawkes, 1996). Women are still expected to subscribe to gendered-age norms and to "act their age" (Ginn & Arber, 2002, p. 8). This exclusion is particularly salient when considered against the background of findings that indicate that men and women alike view sex in later life as an important means of expressing love and facilitating a close emotional relationship. Gott and Hinchliff (2003) found that sex remains an important component of the quality of life as long as people think they can have a sexual partner during their lifetime. Similarly, Muhlbauer and Zemach (1991) reported that being part of a stable intimate relationship enhances the sense of happiness and overall life satisfaction of people at all ages.

The cohort of women now over 50 reached their sexual prime after the sexual revolution. They are, in fact, the first generation that has made the transition to midlife to be sexually defined by a liberal permissive message (Laumann et al., 1994). Consequently, their current sexual attitudes and behaviors can only be understood within this sociohistorical context (Gott & Hinchlilff, 2003). In view of what we have seen above, therefore, women over 50 tend to be caught between often ridiculously absurd, restrictive sexual norms related to middle-aged and elderly women, on the one hand, and their own sexual identity shaped during early adulthood, on the other (Pearlman, 1993). As a result, the transition to middle and later life negatively affects their sexual identity, generates an acute sense of vulnerability and rejection, and thus influences their lifestyle options and well-being in a different manner than it did previous generations.

Age Identity, Social–Historical Development, and Well-being

Whereas the feminist movement and sexual revolution coincided with the early adulthood of today's over 50 cohort, the change of perspectives on middle and old age is still a work in progress. At the heart of the current debate are issues related to the meanings attached to middle age in general and to middle-aged women in particular (Arber & Ginn, 2002). As we have seen, social constructionists reject the view that aging is simply a biological process and argue that it is largely molded by sociocultural factors (Blaikie, 1999). A model proposed by Berger and Luckmann (1991) demonstrates how cultural creations such as aging become actual realities and, in time, are conceived to be natural. These realities are then absorbed by the targeted age group. This is not to say that cultural assumptions regarding old age (or any other social construct) are accepted uncritically. On the contrary, each generation carves out its own meanings for the sets of values specific to its historical period. Indeed, Hirshbein (2001) showed how the cultural meanings of growing old tend to change for different cohorts, and suggested that conceptions of old age will probably continue to be modified as the experience of middle and old age changes.

One of the basic tenets underlying the current debate on aging relates to the specific nature of the experiences of those now in mid- and later life. There is general agreement that the age group that grew up following the Second World War had very different life course experiences than earlier generations (Arber et al., 2003). This is particularly true for the women, who matured at the time of the gender role transformation sparked by the feminist movement and sexual revolution. As there was less pressure on them to base their identities on traditional family roles and relationships, these women experienced, already in young adulthood, multiple roles that reflect a far more balanced gender role composite than ever before. The early experience of multiple roles, according to Vandewater et al. (1997), shapes personality in ways that, later in life, lay the basis for satisfying middle years. The researchers reported that the number of roles at age 28 predicted identity achievement at age 43, which in turn predicted role quality and diversity at age 48. It is these "new" identities of middle-aged women and the ways in which they differ from those of previous cohorts that are capturing the interest of both researchers and the general public. And, whenever the emphasis is on the reconstruction of gendered-age identities, drawn from an extensive repertoire of largely diversified adult roles, it tends to be associated with enhanced well-being.

One of the outcomes of the current change of perspectives on middle and old age is a shift in the dividing lines between age groups and the deconstruction of age group norms and expectations. In some cases, differences within the same age group may be greater than those between different age groups. This greater fluidity of lifestyles across age group boundaries was addressed by Tessa Jowell, the British Secretary for Cultural Affairs, in an interview published in the electronic form of the *Guardian* (Hinsliff, 2004). Jowell claimed that modern older women were no longer easily pigeonholed: "Some of them are themselves bringing up relatively young children, some are already deep into grandmotherhood. Some are still working while others have taken early retirement," and she added that the British Labor Party has not engaged enough with the particular interests of these women because it's so hard to pin them down. She admitted that the party was not really ready for the change that has taken place among women in this age group and that an understanding of the trends and issues is necessary in order to appeal to midlife women's needs and inclinations. The need to update the categorization of age groups was also central to a discussion led by Kaufman (2000) at Cornell University, where it was concluded that what is considered old age has changed dramatically over the last few decades as a function of culture and context.

The importance of age as a regulator of sequentially related life events that mark differences between age groups has thus waned. In other words, the phenomenon defined by developmental theorist Neugarten (1968) as the "social clock" (i.e., socially constructed expectations for organizing one's major events in life [such as marriage, parenthood, retirement] according to accepted age norms) is, to a large extent, obsolete. Consequently, the exclusively vertical stratification of society may soon be replaced, at least in some respects, by a horizontal stratification, thereby doing away with the segmental nature of age groups. Indeed, a more complex combination of physical, social, and psychological parameters would probably be a better and more accurate indicator of a person's lifestyle and well-being.

Outdated Gendered-age Identities and Lifestyles in the Popular Media: Are Those in Their 50s the New Swinging Generation?

Contemporary popular culture, as presented in the media, has an enormous effect on people's lives. Postmodern theorists claim that its power lies in the fact that it effaces the distinction between real and unreal. Strinati (1995), for instance, contended that, "media images increasingly dominate our sense of reality and the way we define ourselves" (p. 224). In this respect, the media play a major role in the ongoing process of socialization, where issues of selection of gender roles and representations are so important. Recent attention has been focused particularly on the cultural status of women (Peach, 1998), and has revealed an interesting development in the evolving sociocultural reality of women in their 50s as reflected in the popular media: an emphasis on the "new identities" of this age group. The mainstream movie *Calendar Girls*, for example, defies the long-standing conviction that a woman's essence and attractiveness are tied to youthfulness. The film shows women over 50 posing nude for a calendar in order to raise money for a charitable cause, clearly enjoying every minute of the experience, and thus challenging the age-old image of midlife and older women as asexual beings. Similarly, the artist Matzkin (2003) produced, and exposed on her website, a series of acrylic portraits of *Naked Old Ladies*, using models aged 58 to 87 in all their "sagging glory," seeking to show that there is beauty in the female form, no matter what age or shape it is. The taboos surrounding nudity in older women have also been broken by commercial firms such as Benetton. A Benetton advertisement in October 2001 in honor of the UN Year of the Volunteer featured a retired German photographer living in California at her local nudist colony, and a high quality version of the advertisement was uploaded onto Benetton's website. In the same year, Ikea used photographs of naked elderly women in magazine ads and billboards in select cities. Popular culture thus appears to be playing up the desirability and attractiveness of women over 50, a trend that is likely to have a positive affect on this generation's self-image.

Another issue being tackled in the mass media, mainly in films, is the persistence of the libido or sexual desires of older women. The British film *The Mother* tells the story of a widow who flirts with her daughter's lover; the death of her husband had awakened her long-suppressed craving for a meaningful and sexually fulfilling relationship. Research on sex and the elderly (Demeter, n.d.) indicates that women are *expected* to become asexual earlier than men are. Women's real-life difficulties, therefore, largely involve cultural myths and unfavorable public attitudes, rather than a diminished sex drive or functioning.

Liberal lifestyles are already emerging in some retirement communities in Denmark, where the elderly residents can choose to watch pornographic videos in the communal television area or to receive regular visits from prostitutes. As one residence manager explained: "Like all other homes we have a council of residents. If they decide that they want to watch porn films in the main living room once a week, we will do it ... We do not reject any suggestion" (www.ananova.com). In a similar vein, an article in the *Washington Post* (Nicolosi, 2001) about the sex lives of older single heterosexuals was accompanied by an extensive list of safe sex tips and resources.

Still, for many older heterosexual women, feeling sexy and having the know-how and capability to engage in a sexual relationship in later life has not necessarily opened up the option of an active sex-life. The greatest barrier was—and remains—the lack of available male partners. The statistics are commonplace: Older men have much more opportunity to engage in intimate relationships, and their partners tend to be considerably younger than they are. However, popular culture, and the film industry in particular, is beginning to question the common beliefs regarding desirable heterosexual matches between mid-life adults. A romantic comedy entitled *Something's Gotta Give*, which featured Diane Keaton and Jack Nicholson, tells the story of the romance and physical attraction between two middle-aged adults. The heroine, a divorced playwright, outstrips the younger competition and enjoys a romantic encounter in Paris. Applauding the preference for same age sexual partners in midlife and later might ultimately create opportunities for older women to practice their sexuality actively.

Newspapers and Internet forums contain references to an additional change in the attitude and behaviors of women in midlife. Ashton and Asthana (2004) reported that a growing number of women are choosing to disregard the stigma of becoming a mother later in life: Pregnancy rates for women over 40 rose by 41%

in the 1990s. They noted that the trend is particularly apparent among celebrities (the "trendsetters"), and quoted their interviewees as saying that the decision to become a parent has to be made in light of many factors, of which age is only one.

It is surprising that so little has been written in the academic literature on the current deconstructionist trends in media representations of women over 50 and their possible implications for enhancing the quality of life of this age group. As previously noted, the media possess enormous power in enmeshing what is real and unreal (Berger & Luckmann, 1991). Thus, the recent cultural images that indicate a gradual shift in cohort-based norms, accentuating new options, particularly in the realm of sexuality and intimate relations, could possibly undermine the exclusivity of traditional conventions related to sex appeal and romance. This development has special significance for women whose perceptions of their own sexuality were established by the liberal messages of the sexual revolution. In this respect, the media representations of role models defying traditional conventions that link women's attractiveness to their youthfulness, might open the way to real life experiences for women over 50. It is worth noting that many of the screen plays of sexual encounters and romantic attachments are portrayed together with experiences and gestures of mastery, personal power, and the willingness to make daring lifestyle choices, all of which are connected with various dimensions of well-being.

The Contractive View

Constraints related to the sexuality, sexual desirability, and sexual activity of women in midlife adversely affect their sense of well-being (Aber et al., 2003). This disadvantage is especially conspicuous in the contemporary sexualized culture of youth. The seemingly commonsense truism that women (and men) do not undergo an instant transformation when they cross the boundary into the 50 age bracket seems unable to hold its own against the prevalent traditional perceptions of normative sex appeal and age-appropriate sexual activity. The cohort of women now in their 50s is, therefore, beset by tensions between what they experience as psychological and physiological needs and the socio-cultural constraints on the realization of those needs. As these issues are addressed more thoroughly in this volume by Joan Chrisler and by Maureen McHugh, I will limit myself to only a few brief remarks on the subject.

As we have seen, assessment of the well-being of the present cohort of women over 50 takes into account the sweeping sociocultural changes in gendered-age roles in the last four decades. The social constructionist orientation advances the notion that many gender and age differences are conditioned by social context and thus tend to change in different generations (Stewart & Ostrove, 1998). Having absorbed values and behavioral codes associated with the feminist movement and the sexual revolution, women over 50 now feel "young at heart." Indeed, Ryff (1991) found a resemblance between young and middle-aged adults on all dimensions of well-being, and both groups expected continued gains in the years ahead. This may be one explanation for the resentment and fear experienced by older women in the face of sexual constraints and losses.

The concept of "possible selves" introduced by Markus and Nurius (1986) is also helpful in addressing the difficulties of midlife women with respect to sexuality. Possible selves are defined as the "cognitive components of hopes, fears, goals, and threats" (p. 954). Women who were exposed to liberal sexual messages in young adulthood have incorporated them into their structure of accessible and desirable selves. Frustration is only to be expected when they are rather suddenly confronted with cultural barriers that exclude the sexual self from the range of possible selves.

The fact that, at present, the feelings and expectations of women in midlife are not supported by the dominant social norms and cultural representations is indicative of what Davidson and Fennel (2002, p. 4) referred to as a "cultural lag" (i.e., cultural conceptions have not caught up with the changes in the way women experience their sexuality in reality and their expectation of acting accordingly). However, as indicated above, at least some of the popular media allow open, sometimes even subversive, discourse on sexual ethics and fresh cultural representations of the body, sex appeal, and sexual activity of middle-aged women. Future studies are needed to examine the interaction between what remain the separate expansive and contractive domains of well-being and the quality of life of women over 50.

Conclusions

I have focused here on the well-being of women in their 50s from a sociocultural perspective, highlighting the favorable effect of cultural shifts in social constructs, such as gender and age. Middle-aged women today tend to score similarly to younger women on well-being assessment scales, partly because they tend to retain the liberal values and empowered behavioral codes acquired in young adulthood. In this sense, they differ not only from older women, but also from middle-aged women in previous generations. The latter difference can be explained by the social constructionist orientation: It is connected to changes in structural opportunities, mainly in education and employment, as well as to shifts in the normative expectations concerning gender and age roles (Parker & Aldwin, 1997). In other words, the expansion and growth in well-being that have been found in recent years for women in this age group are related to an increase in the available personal resources (and/or to the decrease in the personal constraints) that can be expected at this stage in life (according to the developmental perspective), along with sometimes dramatic advances in cultural representations and opportunities.

It stands to reason that the major shifts in the balance of power in society in the last four decades, often reflected in gender and age crossovers or in a blurring of demarcation lines between groups, have facilitated this change. Women in their 50s have more power today than ever before, and consequently display better positive functioning (as defined by current theories, e.g., Keyes et al., 2002; Ryff & Keyes, 1995). This leads us to question the connection between structures of well-being and power constructs, both on the personal and the institutional levels. Indeed, well-being appears to have significant political implications as well as personal ones.

Nevertheless, the literature on issues such as the physical attraction and sexual activity of middle-aged women reveals a totally different perspective. The culture still delimits normative desirability and sexual relations. Thus, women in their 50s are seen as empowered and admirable, but not necessarily desirable. As a result, side by side with enhanced positive well-being (Ryff & Keyes 1995), an increase in adverse psychological responses (e.g., vulnerability, anxiety, frustration, loneliness) has been found (Gott & Hinchliff, 2003). Thus, the culturally segmented representations of women in midlife may very well account for their fragmented structures of well-being.

However, the story of women currently in midlife is still being written. These women are bringing a new understanding of sexuality and intimate relationships based on perceptions of their own sexual needs and preferences. They also seem to be taking an active role in re-conceptualizing intimate relations and experimenting with new forms of togetherness such as living apart together (Borell & Karlsson, 2003). Thus, although it cannot be concluded that the socio-cultural constraints concerning sex appeal and intimate attachments that beset women in midlife are soon to be washed away, it seems feasible to speculate that the quality of their lives might still be markedly improved.

References

Arber, S., and Ginn, J. (Eds.). (2002). *Connecting gender and ageing: A sociological approach.* Buckingham, UK: Open University Press.

Arber, S., Davidson, K., and Ginn, J. (2003). Changing approaches to gender and later life. In S. Arber, K. Davidson, and J. Ginn (Eds.), *Gender and ageing* (pp. 1–15) Maidenhead, UK: Open University Press.

Ashton, L., and Asthana, A. (2004, February 15). Nappies at fifty. Retrieved July13, 2005 from http://www.observer.guardian.co.uk.

Barnett, R.C., and Baruch, G.K. (1978). Women in the middle years: A critique of research and theory. *Psychology of Women Quarterly, 3*, 187–198.

Bart, B.P. (1971). Depression in middle-aged women. In J.M. Bardwick (Ed.), *Readings on the psychology of women* (pp. 134–143). New York: Harper & Row.

Baumeister, R.F. (2000). Gender differences in erotic plasticity: The female sex drive as socially flexible and responsive. *Psychological Bulletin, 126*, 347–374.

Benetton advertisement. (2001, October). Retrieved May, 12, 2004, from *http://www.benetton.com.*

Berger, P., and Luckmann, T. (1991). *The social construction of reality: A treatise in the sociology of knowledge.* Harmondsworth, UK: Penguin. [Original work published in 1966.]

Blaikie, A. (1999). *Ageing and popular culture.* Cambridge: Cambridge University Press.

Borell, K., and Karlsson, S.G. (2003). Re-conceptualizing intimacy and ageing: Living apart together. In S. Arber, K. Davidson and J. Ginn (Eds.), *Gender and ageing* (pp. 1–15) Maidenhead, UK: Open University Press.

Broverman, I.K., Broverman, D.M., Clarkson, F.E., Rosenkrantz, P.S., and Vogel, S.R. (1970). Sex-role stereotypes and clinical judgments of mental health. *Journal of Consulting and Clinical Psychology, 34*, 1–7.
Burns, A., and Leonard, R. (2005). Chapters of our lives: Life narratives of midlife and older Australian women. *Sex Roles, 52*, 269–277.
Cheng, S.T. (2004). Age and subjective well-being revisited: A discrepancy perspective. *Psychology and Aging, 19*, 409–415.
Collins, L.H. (1998). Illustrating feminist theory: Power and psychopathology. *Psychology of Women Quarterly, 22*, 97–112.
Davidson, K., and Fennell, G. (2002). New intimate relationship in later life. *Ageing International, 27*, 3–10.
Demeter, D. (n.d.). Sex and the elderly. Retrieved May 5, 2004, from University of Missouri-Kansas City, The human sexuality web site: *http://www.* umkc.edu\sites\hsw\age.
Denmark, F.L. (1994). Engendering psychology. *American Psychologist, 49*, 329–324.
Ehrenreich, B., Hess, E., and Jacobs, G. (1986). *Re-making love: The feminization of sex.* Garden City, NY: Doubleday Anchor.
Friedman, A. (1996). *Annie Oakley won twice: Intimacy and power in female identity.* Tel-Aviv: Hakibbutz Hameuchad.
Gergen, K.J. (1985). The social constructionist movement in modern psychology. *American Psychologist, 40*, 266–275.
Gergen, M.M. (1990). Finished at 40: Women's development within patriarchy. *Psychology of Women Quarterly, 14*, 471–493.
Ginn, J., and Arber, S. (2002). Only connect: Gender relations and ageing. In S. Arber and J. Ginn (Eds.), *Connecting gender* and *ageing: A sociological approach* (pp. 1–14). Buckingham, UK: Open University Press.
Gott, M., and Hinchliff, S. (2003). Sex and ageing: A gendered issue. In S. Arber, K. Davidson., and J. Ginn (Eds.), *Gender and ageing* (pp. 63–79). Maidenhead, UK: Open University Press.
Gutmann, D. (1975). Parenthood: A key to the comparative study of the life cycle. In N. Datan and L. Ginsberg (Eds.), *Life-span developmental psychology: Normative life crises* (pp. 98–119). San Diego, CA: Academic Press.
Hawkes, G. (1996). *A sociology of sex and sexuality.* Buckingham, UK: Open University Press.
Helgeson, V.S. (1994). Relation of agency and communion to well-being: Evidence and potential explanations. *Psychological Bulletin, 116*, 412–428.
Helson, R. (1997). The self in middle age. In M.E. Lachman and J.B. James (Eds.), *Multiple paths of middle development* (pp. 21–43). Chicago: University of Chicago Press.
Helson, R., and Moane, G. (1987). Personality change in women from college to midlife. *Journal of Social Psychology, 53*, 176–186.
Helson, R., and Picano, J. (1990). Is the traditional role bad for women? *Journal of Personality and Social Psychology, 59*, 311–320.
Helson, R., and Wink, P. (1992). Personality change in women from the early 40s to the early 50s. *Psychology of Aging, 7*, 46–55.
Hinsliff, G. (2004, April 25). The calendar girl generation. Retrieved May 8, 2004, from http://www.guardian.co.uk.
Hirshbein, L.D. (2001). Popular views of old age in America, 1900–1950. *Journal of American Geriatrics Society, 4*, 1555–1560.
Ikea. (2001, October). Retrieved May 5, 2004, from http://www.philly.com. Press.

Kaufman, D. (2000). Sex and the elderly woman. Retrieved May 6, 2004, from www.globalaging.org\health\us.

Kaufman, S.R. (1986). *The ageless self.* Madison, WI: University of Wisconsin Press.

Keyes, C.L.M., Shmotkin, D., and Ryff, C.D. (2002). Optimizing well-being: The empirical encounter of two traditions. *Journal of Personality and Social Psychology, 82*, 1007–1022.

Laumann, E.O., Gagnon, J.H., Michael, R.T., and Michaels, S. (1994). *The social organization of sexuality: Sexual practices in the United States.* Chicago: University of Chicago Press.

Lauzen, M.M., and Dozier, D.M. (2005). Maintaining the double standard: Portrayals of age and gender in popular films. *Sex Roles, 52*, 437–446.

Livson, B.F. (1976). Patterns of personality development in middle-aged women: A longitudinal study. *International Journal of Aging and Human Development, 7*, 107–115.

Livson, B. F (1981). Paths to psychological health in middle years: Sex differences. In D.H. Eichorn, J.A. Clausen, M.P. Honzik, and P. Mussen (Eds.), *Present and past in midlife* (pp. 195–221). San Diego, CA: Academic Press.

Lorber, J. (1994). *Paradoxes of gender.* New Haven, CT: Yale University Press.

Markus, H., and Nurius, P. (1986). Possible selves. *American Psychologist, 41*, 954–969.

Matzkin, A. (2003). The naked body. Retrieved May 10, 2004, from www.matzkinstudio.com.

Mitchell, V., and Helson, R. (1990). Women's prime of life—Is it the 50s?. *Psychology of Women Quarterly, 14*, 451–470.

Mosedale, S. (2005). Assessing women's empowerment: Toward a conceptual framework. *Journal of International Development, 17*, 243–257.

Muhlbauer, V., and Zemach, M. (1991). *Onesies twosies.* Tel Aviv: Am Oved.

Neugarten, B.L. (1968). Adult personality: Toward a psychology of the life cycle. In B.L. Neugarten (Ed.), *Middle age and aging: A reader in social psychology* (pp. 137–147). Chicago: University of Chicago Press.

Neugarten, B.L., and Gutmann, D. (1968). Age sex-roles and personality in middle age: A thematic apperception study. In B L. Neugarten (Ed.), *Middle age and aging: A reader in social psychology* (pp. 77–84). Chicago: University of Chicago Press.

Neugarten, B.L., and Neugarten, D.A. (1996). The changing meanings of age. In D.A. Neugarten (Ed.), *The meaning of age: Selected papers of Bernice L. Neugarten* (pp. 72–77). Chicago: University of Chicago Press.

Nicolosi, M. (July, 2001). Sex lives of older single heterosexuals. Retrieved May, 8 2004, from http://www.washingtonpost.com.

Parker, R.A., and Aldwin, C.J. (1997). Do aspects of gender identity change from early to middle adulthood? Disentangling age, cohort, and period effects. In M.E. Lachman and J.B. James (Eds.), *Multiple paths of middle development* (pp. 67–109). Chicago: University of Chicago Press.

Peach, L.J. (1998). Sex, sexism, sexual harassment, and sexual abuse. In L .J. Peach (Ed.), *Women in culture: A women's studies anthology* (pp. 283–301). Oxford: Blackwell.

Pearlman, S.F. (1993). Late mid-life astonishment: Disruptions to identity and self-esteem. In N.D. Davis., E. Cole., and E.D. Rothblum (Eds.), *Faces of women and aging* (pp. 1–13). New York: Harrington Park Press.

Pietromonaco, P.R., Manis, J., and Frohardt-Lane, K. (1986). Psychological consequences of multiple social roles. *Psychology of Women Quarterly, 10*, 373–382.

Powell, J.L., and Moores, J. (2001). Theorising social gerontology: The case of social philosophies of age. *E-Journal of Culture Studies.* Retrieved 8 June, 2005, from *http://www.*fuentes.csh.udg.mx./cuchs/sincronia.

Rosenkrantz, P., Vogel, S., Bee, H., Broverman, I., and Broverman, D. (1968). Sex role stereotypes and self-concept in college students. *Journal of Consulting Clinical Psychology, 32*, 287–295.

Rossi, A.S. (2004). The menopausal transition and aging processes. In O.G. Brim, C.D. Ryff, and R.C. Kessler (Eds.), *How healthy are we? A national study of well-being at midlife* (pp. 153–201). Chicago: University of Chicago Press.

Ryff, C.D. (1987). The place of personality and social structure research in social psychology. *Journal of Personality and Social Psychology, 53*, 1192–1202.

Ryff, C.D. (1991). Possible selves in adulthood and old age: A tale of shifting horizons. *Psychology and Aging, 6*, 286–295.

Ryff, C.D., and Keyes, C.L.M. (1995). The structure of psychological well-being revisited. *Journal of Personality and Social Psychology, 69*, 719–727.

Ryff, C.D., and Singer, B. (1998). The contours of positive human health. *Psychological Inquiry, 9*, 1–28.

Schmuck, P., and Sheldon, K.M. (2001). Life goals and well-being: To the frontiers of life goal research. In P. Schmuck and K.M. Sheldon (Eds.), *Life goals and well-being* (pp. 1–17). Seattle: Hogrefe and Huber.

Schmutte, P.S., and Ryff, C.D. (1997). Personality and well-being: Reexamining methods and meanings. *Journal of Personality and Social Psychology, 73*, 549–559.

Stewart, A., and Healy, J.M. (1989). Linking individual development and social changes. *American Psychologist, 44*, 30–42.

Stewart, A.J., and Ostrove, J.M. (1998). Women's personality in middle age: Gender, history, and midcourse corrections. *American Psychologist, 53*, 1185–1194.

Strinati, D. (1995). *An introduction to theories of popular culture*. London: Routledge.

Thoits, P.A. (1983). Multiple theories and psychological well-being: A reformulation and test of the social isolation hypothesis. *American Sociological Review, 48*, 174–187.

Thoits, P.A. (2003). Personal agency in the accumulation of multiple role-identities. In P.J. Burke, T.J. Owens, R.T. Serpe, and P.A. Thoits (Eds.), *Advances in identity theory and research* (pp. 179–194). New York: Kluwer Academic/Plenum.

Vandewater, E.A., Ostrove, J.M., and Stewart, A.J. (1997). Predicting women's well-being in midlife: The importance of personality development and social role involvements. *Journal of Personality and Social Psychology, 72*, 1147–1160.

Welsh, W.M., and Stewart, A.J. (1995). Relationship between women and their parents: Implications for midlife well-being. *Psychology and Aging, 10*, 181–190.

Wolf, N. (1998). The beauty myth. In L.J. Peach (Ed.), *Women in culture* (pp. 179–187). Oxford: Blackwell.

Woodhill, B.M., and Samuels, C.A. (2003). Positive and negative androgyny and their relationship with psychological health and well-being. *Sex Roles, 48*, 555–567.

6
Enjoying the Returns: Women's Friendships After 50

Suzanna M. Rose

Women after 50 show a new vigor in their friendships. The second half of life elicits review and contemplation concerning where one has been and also, sometimes, decision and change concerning the personal priorities that will guide the remaining decades. New perspectives of the self and intimacy emerge. As time becomes more valuable, choices about how and with whom to spend it become more pressing. As women assess their lives, they also take stock of their friendships, often making deliberate and clear-eyed decisions about where to increase and reduce their emotional investment. Old friendships may be recalibrated or new ones sought to match fresh views of the self and relationships. What does not change is the immense importance women attach to their friendships. Commitment to the role of friend is even more predictive than income or marital status in the determination of older women's life satisfaction (Trotman & Brody, 2002).

In this chapter, the expectations, functions, and development of women's friendships after age 50 will be hypothesized and explored. This is relatively new terrain from the standpoint of psychological research, which has focused on friendship among the young or old but given little attention to the middle years. Thus, speculation will be required. Factors that typically are known to affect friendship will be considered as well, including historical forces, gender, sexual orientation, race and ethnicity, individual differences, and culture. Negative aspects of friendship such as conflict and false friends also will be discussed. Fruitful research directions will be proposed to begin a systematic exploration of women's friendships after age 50.

Historical Influences on Friendship

Current views of women's friendship contrast sharply with those that prevailed a century ago and until the recent past. At present, women's friendships with other women are regarded as a psychological asset that contributes to happiness, health, and well-being. A large amount of well-being research documents the finding that women's same-sex friendships are more intimate and supportive than men's (Bank & Hansford, 2003). Women tend to enjoy same-sex friendships more than men do because of the greater intimacy between women friends (e.g., Bank, 1995).

In contrast, the dominant view from the time of Aristotle until the 1970s was that women were incapable of true friendship. One argument was that women were not genetically programmed to bond with one another; others asserted that sexual jealousy and the desire for men's approval inevitably resulted in hostility between women that prevented friendship. Women's friendships often were trivialized as being "two-faced," "gossipy," or "juvenile" (O'Connor, 1992).

With the growth of women's studies and also the "science of relationships" from the 1970s to the mid-1980s, more positive attention was focused on women's friendship. Contextual factors that affect women's friendships were emphasized. For instance, the primacy of marriage as a social institution, particularly for women, was recognized as lessening opportunities for friendship (O'Connor, 1992). Feminist historians also challenged the negative view of women's friendships by uncovering numerous cases of romantic friendship between women friends during the 1800s (e.g., Faderman, 1981). However, the research that resulted from those analyses was aimed primarily at identifying gender differences rather than understanding the nature of women's friendship in its own right. Thus, women's friendships continued to be regarded as secondary attachments relative to the marital bond, a view that reflects implicit heterosexist and patriarchal views of the importance of women's friendship (Rose, 2000).

A more recent trend has emerged that questions the secondary status of women's friendship. For instance, the emotional strength of women's friendships was found to be no different from their relationships with husbands or lovers (Goodenow & Gaier, 1990). Women's longer lifespan in the developed countries and the likelihood that they will outlive their husbands has resulted in reconsiderations of the importance of friendship, particularly later in life (Allan, 2001). This new interest in women's friendship highlights the fact that very little is known about this important relationship, particularly during midlife. Much more remains to be explored concerning the convergence of life stage and friendship for women after 50.

Expectations of Friends

Expectations of friends in Western, industrialized cultures tend to be idealized. Friendships typically are expected to involve intimacy, enjoyment, dependability, acceptance, and caring. Furthermore, women's expectations for friendship tend to be very high. Gouldner and Strong (1987) reported that the middle-aged women in their study expressed "a great longing for friendship" and described their idealized friendships in terms that were similar to those used for romantic relationships:

The perfect friend was thought of as possessing, above all, the traits of trustworthiness and unswerving loyalty and the ability to keep confidences. She was a person, who was, at the same time, a good listener, an entertaining companion, someone with whom she could gossip and air serious problems. Ideally she would provide sympathy and opportunities for catharsis and self-insight along with distraction and fun. (p. 105)

The "voluntariness" of friendship contributes to its idealized status as well as distinguishes it from other social relations. Unlike marital or family relationships that are bound by institutional ties, friendships are chosen. They are not facilitated by social roles and are not coerced. Other characteristics unique to friendship include autonomy, sentiment, and freedom from structural constraints. In addition, friendships tend to be governed by the norms of reciprocity and equality. These features lend themselves to popular conceptions of friendship as private, self-governing dyads that are voluntary and informal (Bell & Coleman, 1999).

It is not known if women's friendships at midlife diverge from the descriptions above. Although midlife women may wish for the ideal, there is reason to believe they may be more appreciative of authenticity in themselves and others that could lead to greater tolerance for the foibles and failings of friends and self. On the other hand, as awareness of death becomes more salient to women in their 50s, they may desire to break free from scripted roles, discover new or rejected aspects of the self, or seek a greater sense of wholeness. The feeling that the time is "now or never" to do something meaningful can impact friendships negatively if friends want to maintain the status quo.

Friendship Functions

Adults of all ages endorse six functions of friendships (Argyle & Henderson, 1984). At a minimum, friends are supposed to stand up for each other (even in a friend's absence), share news of success, provide emotional support, trust and confide in each other, volunteer help when needed, and try to make the friend happy when together. In addition, close friends are supposed to repay debts and favors, be tolerant of the friend's other friends, avoid criticizing the friend in public, keep confidences, avoid jealousy and criticism of other relationships, avoid nagging, and respect privacy. Violation of these functions is likely to jeopardize the friendship.

Friendships play a unique and crucial role in adults' lives. Friends' similarity in terms of personal and lifestyle characteristics makes them well suited to affirm each other's identity, reminisce, give advice, provide socialization, share leisure activities, and help with nontechnical tasks. Friends are expected to provide the companionship and emotional support required to meet the losses and transitions of growing older.

Equality is a distinguishing feature of friendship. Friends are happiest when the friendship is perceived as being equal in terms of the "give-and-take" in the relationship (Roberto, 2001). Inequalities in material resources or interpersonal power must be leveled between friends or the friendship may not survive. Reciprocity also is important, particularly in the early stages. Established friendships are expected to be "communal" rather than "exchange" relationships (Clark & Mills, 1993). Communal relations do not require that a specific debt be returned with a comparable benefit, as would be expected in exchange relationships. Equality of affect rather than equality of exchange governs communal relations.

Long-term friends provide a sense of continuity with the past, and over time they may be regarded as family, which enhances a sense of connectedness (Lewittes, 1989). Women (and men) report being happier spending time with friends than with anyone else (Larson & Bradney, 1988). Fortunately, friendships among older women contribute to psychological growth, as well as to physical and mental health (Patrick et al., 2001).

Gender Roles

Friendships are strongly affected by gender roles. Women are more likely to provide solace, sympathy, and sophisticated types of emotional support to their friends than men are (e.g., Basow & Rubenfeld, 2003). These behaviors are learned early in life. Girls are encouraged much more than boys to behave in a nurturing way toward others, to talk about their emotions, and to express sympathy. By adulthood, women are not only better at giving nurturance and support, they are *expected* to be ready and willing to provide it.

Women place a high premium on giving and receiving comfort from their friends, which suggests that women who are unable to provide it will be negatively perceived or rejected (Holmstrom et al., 2005). Although gender roles are robust across the lifespan, countervailing forces at midlife might temper stereotypic expectations for unconditional support from women friends. Anecdotal evidence suggests that women in midlife come to value truth-telling more than they did when they were young. Levine (2005) characterized this as a "new intimacy": "We are much more forthcoming about our failings and failures, more willing to seek and accept advice, less know-it-all about dispensing advice, and a lot less concerned with eliciting sympathy for its own sake" (p. 145). The expectation for a greater level of honesty may free women to have a greater range of response to friends' predicaments. Less sympathy and more direct advice, such as "don't be upset about that" or "you'd better get your act together," might be given and appreciated.

The Development of Friendship

The usual path to friendship is for women of similar attitudes, activities, and social class standing to meet and become friends as their paths cross frequently (Fehr, 1996). The connection at first may be superficial and based on an "even exchange" of pleasantries, invitations, or activities. Over time, if the interest is mutual, a gradual transition through a series of increasingly intimate, personal disclosures will occur and lead to a closer friendship. As trust and self-disclosure increase, the friendship becomes based more on communal norms such as mutual concern than on a formal reciprocity regarding what one gives or gets in the friendship (Clark & Mills, 1993).

Making Friends

The formation of friendship is constrained by at least three factors that affect the opportunities adults have to meet potential friends and promote friendship. First, demographic variables tend to limit friendship. At all ages, women tend to come into contact with women who are similar in terms of age, race, social class, sexual orientation, and who live and work in similar areas. Women with young children often become friends with mothers of their children's friends. Roberto (2001) reported that older women tend to live close to their close friends, to be about the same age and social class status, and to share social and ethnic backgrounds.

Second, the norm of equality in friendship also tends to restrain the development of friendships across socioeconomic status or identity categories that cause social distance. For instance, a friendship between a woman and her household worker must surmount both economic barriers and social ones caused by inequality of rank in the social order. Similarly, friendships between Black and White women or lesbians and heterosexual women may have to meet additional criteria in order to bridge the social distance and to put the friendship on an equal footing (e.g., Hall & Rose, 1996).

Patriarchal definitions of women's place as secondary and subservient to men also shape women's friendships. Among heterosexual couples, men's preferences and friendships often dictate couples' social lives. Women more often than men report that dating or marriage precipitates the loss of a same-sex friendship (Gullestad, 1984; Rose, 1984). Wives may seek to maintain friendships with their women friends independent of their husbands, but arranging to see women friends separately from couple activities requires extra effort and makes the friendships more difficult to maintain. The negative effect of marriage on women's friendships continues after divorce or widowhood. Both divorced and widowed women report having to rebuild their friendship networks (e.g., Armstrong & Goldsteen, 1990). Once the husband is no longer present, his friends may drop the wife as a friend.

Situational factors that arise from male dominance and gender roles also place major constraints on women's friendships. As Enright and Rawlinson (1992) pointed out: "The bosom of the family is not a rich breeding ground for friendships" (p. 96). Women continue to shoulder about 70% of the household and child care responsibilities, and most have little free time for their own leisure pursuits (e.g., Green et al., 1990). Women earn less than men on average and have fewer resources to use in establishing and maintaining friendships. Women also have less access to and less control of public space than men do, including parks, bars, social clubs, athletic courts, and arcades. Fear of violence from men limits women's forays alone outside the home. Thus, demographic, social, and physical constraints limit friendship choice and interactions.

By age 50, some of the limitations on women's friendships described above may be reduced. Working women in their 50s are more likely to have their own financial resources and also to have more leisure time due to a decline in family and household responsibilities as children grow up and leave home. In fact, the 50s might amount to a "golden age" of women's friendships, given that women are likely to be at their height of confident power (i.e., Neugarten, 1968), financial stability, and still in relatively good health. It may be the era when women fully learn to "treat a friendship like the gift that it is" (Paul, 2004, p. 164).

Maintaining Friendships

Studies of friendship in the middle years have not asked about the strategies used to maintain friendships. Friends interact both at home and in community activities. Getting together to talk is the most common social activity, but friends also help each other with transportation, shopping, and running errands (Adams, 1997). Communication strategies are important in friendship maintenance throughout life. Aspects of communication that create tension are the interplay between independence and dependence in friendship and between friendship's protective and expressive functions. Friendships provide room for women to pursue individual goals and interests, but also in times of need require interdependence. These two privileges of friendship require ongoing negotiations to keep the friendship in balance. Likewise, friends must balance expressiveness with protectiveness. Honesty, candor, and self-disclosure have to be managed carefully to avoid harming the friend.

Ending Friendships

Friendships may end for a number of reasons, but this has been examined empirically in only a few studies of either younger or older adults. Causes of endings cited by women and men in their 20s included lack of social skills or reciprocity, inappropriate self-disclosures, inability to express feelings, and learning something distasteful about the friend (e.g., Rose, 1984). Women are more likely than men to lose a friendship because their romantic relationship competed with the friendship for time. Adults in their mid-20s to mid-30s attributed friendship endings to a lack of respect for privacy and too much demand for personal advice (Argyle & Henderson, 1984). In old age, active termination of friendship is rarely reported other than due to the death of a friend. Friendships either decline or end by "fading away" due to a change in lifestyle or pathway over the years, a move, or major breaches of friendship norms (Bleiszner & Adams, 1992).

At present, no research exists that addresses how and when midlife women end friendships. However, developmental research concerning women at midlife suggests that they may act to terminate even long-term friendships if they are chronically unsatisfying. For instance, Gersick and Kram (2002) studied high achieving professional women at midlife and reported that the age 50 transition was characterized by the task of coming into one's own. This task deals with gaining confidence in one's abilities, knowing what one wants, and being able to go after it. The women's stories suggested that a wellspring of energy to pursue one's own life was released during the age 50 transition. The reassessment of relationships during this period, combined with increased confidence to ask for what one wants, hypothetically might trigger decisions to end unsatisfying friendships.

For example, one woman approaching 50 who had recently ended a 25-year-old friendship described it this way: "The older you get, the wiser you get about your own personality and what you're willing to compromise. You become more selective. You're not going to waste time on people who don't share common goals in friendship. If you have a friend who just takes, forget about it! If you're in a friendship where you are just giving, giving, giving, you're going to burn out. In a long distance friendship, it may take years for the animosity to build. That's what happened with Lois" (personal communication, 2006). The dissatisfaction in this friendship stemmed from a lack of reciprocity in visiting each other and in showing interest in the friend's life and relationships.

At midlife, the extent to which gender differences occur in response to troubled or lost friendships is unknown. Women have a better history of making and maintaining friendships throughout life than do men. As women age, they may be less upset than men if friendships end because they are more likely to establish new ones. Or, women's self-concept in later life may be less entangled with the need to perform well at relationships. It remains to be determined if gender differences in response to friendship problems or endings may disappear or even reverse after age 50.

The Diversity of Friendship

Almost all research on friendship has been done on White, middle class women in the United States, particularly young, White college students. Thus, only a little is known about the lives or friendships of Women of Color, lesbians, or working class, poor, or wealthy women. The few studies available provide some limited insights concerning some variables that may affect midlife women's friendship.

Race and Ethnicity

Research on Black women suggests that they may have somewhat different expectations for friendship and that family roles may conflict with friendships. For instance, women place a high premium on giving and receiving sympathy from their friends, but this may be truer of White women than of Black women. Research with college students (White and Black) indicates that women who were unsympathetic helpers to other women were judged as less likeable by other women than were men who were similarly unsympathetic (Holmstrom et al., 2005). Young Black women proved to be an exception to this rule; they found messages that were classified as "cold comfort" by White women, such as giving advice, to be more sensitive and effective.

Other research also indicates that Blacks value the ability to express rather than to repress emotions, and they may adopt a style in friendship that is intense, outspoken, forward, and assertive (Samter et al., 1997). Young Asian American women also perceived highly person-centered comforting strategies in friendship as significantly less sensitive and effective than did White women (Samter et al., 1997). As yet, no research has been done to determine if these expectations apply to women over 50 from various ethnic groups. However, previous research with younger women suggests that cross race friendships between Black, Asian, and White women may be problematic, if White women expect sympathy and Black and Asian women do not.

The division of household labor has been found to affect life satisfaction among Black women, and, by extrapolation, it might also affect friendship. Tangri et al. (2003) studied college-educated Black women at midlife and reported that their personal satisfaction with their lives was influenced by household burden. Household burden refers to the inequitable division of labor within the home. Those with less household burden reported more satisfaction. One might speculate that household burden is inversely related to time to spend with friends. Thus, household burden might be an important variable to include in studies of Black women's midlife friendships.

Core values of various ethnic groups also may have a significant impact on friendship. These are just beginning to be explored. For instance, Latinas/os place a high value on turning to the family for support instead of seeking external help from friends, coworkers, and neighbors, even when the family is acculturated to life in the United States (Keefe et al., 1979). However, young Latina college women were found to rely more on friends than family in order to cope with academic and social stress (Rodriguez et al., 2003). It may be that midlife Latinas also would experience a discrepancy between ethnic group expectations and the norms of the dominant culture, but that remains in question.

Social Class and Friendship

Social class strongly influences women's friendships. First, patterns of forming friendship differ by social class. The middle class pattern for making friends involves broadening the context in which the interaction occurs. For example, this means that a friendly acquaintance from a yoga class might be invited to dinner at the other's home. The relationship then becomes defined not by the specific context (i.e., an exercise class) but would be broadened in a way that emphasized the primacy of the relationship over the original context (Allan, 1998).

Working class friendships tend to be organized differently. The context and setting are emphasized more, and the significance of the tie in its own right is underplayed (Allan, 1998). Friendships tend to stay bounded within the initial context, for example, a church group, and are more dependent on joint participation in those specific activities. Thus, working class relations might not as easily be classified as friendships, because cultural definitions of friendship define it as a relationship that exists outside of specific contexts.

Friendship maintenance among working class women relies mainly on informal mutual aid (Greenberg & Motenko, 1994). Typically, working class families rely more on primary kin living nearby to provide day-to-day support, and they may have relatively few people whom they would name as friends (Allan, 1998). In contrast, middle class women interact with friends more often, provide more assistance to their friends, and are more satisfied with the support they receive in turn (Krause & Borawski-Clark, 1995). In fact, friendships play a larger role in the lives of middle class individuals than kin do (Allan, 1998). The greater mobility of middle class women may result in having fewer kin nearby, which causes greater reliance on friends.

Friendships across social classes are often difficult to establish and maintain. The difference described above between working class and middle class norms is one barrier. Social class also impinges on equality in a friendship. Friends are expected to regard and treat each other as social equals. Difference can be tolerated if it does not undermine the sense that each person has equal social worth. Reciprocity also is expected in friendship, although exchanges do not have to be in-kind and do not have to be returned immediately. However, if two women have unequal or limited resources, the balance of equal social worth and reciprocity is upset (Allan, 1998). For instance, working class women may not have the resources to entertain at home or to dine at restaurants as middle class women may be able to do.

For women at midlife, social class norms are likely to be entrenched. This suggests that working class women after 50 would be more embedded in kin networks than would middle class women. In contrast, middle class women may be freer to cultivate friendships at midlife than ever before. As a result, midlife friendships across social class may be unlikely.

Lesbian Friendships at Midlife

Lesbian friendships are another understudied area. Friendships for lesbians are often the main, if not sole, source of affirmation, support, and love (Stanley, 1996). Friends may take on greater importance to lesbians than to heterosexual women because friends may become surrogate families, replacing kin networks that have rejected them (Weinstock, 2000). At midlife, friendships play an important role for lesbians. Tully (1989) studied a sample of mostly White, professional, midlife lesbians and reported that women friends were identified as the people from whom the most social support was sought and received. Many older lesbians maintain a supportive network of friendships that is fueled by the high value lesbians place on friendship (Weinstock, 2000). Midlife lesbians tend to spend time with and receive support from other lesbians their own age, including lovers, ex-lovers, and friends (e.g., Bradford & Ryan, 1991; Sang, 1991). Rothblum et al. (1995) noted that midlife may bring with it a renewed sense of the importance of friends, particularly because lesbians may not anticipate finding sufficient support from formal caregiving service systems as they age.

Ex-lovers are a significant source of friendship among lesbians, particularly at midlife (Weinstock, 2004). Weeks et al. (2001) and Weston (1997) found that lesbians often included their ex-lovers, as well as their current lovers, as part of their close circle of friends. Lesbians were twice as likely as gay men to report that their best friend was a former lover (Nardi & Sherrod, 1994) and also twice as likely as heterosexual women to report being close to their ex-lovers (Fertitta, 1994, as cited in Kimmel & Sang, 1995). This is far from the norm in heterosexual relations, where friendships between ex-spouses are unusual and, until recently, have been regarded as evidence of "dysfunctional dependency" (Masheter, 1997).

Lesbian friendships raise questions concerning the nature of friendship and hidden assumptions in previous research. The lifelong and central importance lesbians attribute to friendship contests the idea that friendships are "secondary attachments" and challenges heterosexist assumptions that denigrate women's friendships relative to heterosexual love relationships. For instance, Kitzinger (1996) remarked that language often trivializes friendships: "If a sexual relationship is a 'primary relationship,' does this mean that friendships are 'secondary'? If a sexual partner is a 'significant other,' are friendships 'insignificant others'? And what about the question, 'Are you two together, or are you just friends?' when we are both 'together' and 'friends' and there is no 'just' about it"? (p. 296). Perhaps most important, midlife lesbian friendships suggest that more might be gained by studying friendships that have not been limited by the sexist constraints on women's affection that have been imposed on heterosexual women's friendships.

Individual Differences

Any discussion of friendship must take individual differences into account. Women have different personalities and may not approach friendship in the same way. Three elements of adult personality development that might affect friendships are identity, generativity, and confident power (Stewart et al., 2001). Research indicates that identity development is positively related to self-esteem and life satisfaction in midlife women and that the early attainment of a well-articulated identity also is related to women's well-being at midlife (Vandeventer et al., 1997). Generativity refers to the second stage of adulthood posited by Erikson (1968). In generativity, "a man and a woman must have defined for themselves what and whom they have come to care for, what they care to do well, and how they plan to take care of what they have started and created" (Erikson, 1968, p. 395). If this stage is not mastered, the negative outcome is stagnation. A third element of personality at midlife is confident power. Neugarten (1968) proposed that executive processes such as mastery and competence make up the core of the middle-aged personality. Research confirms that middle-aged women feel more in command of their world and themselves than do adults of other ages (e.g., Cartwright & Wink, 1994). Specifically, women report increases in confidence, dominance, and coping skills from early adulthood to middle age (e.g., Stewart et al., 2001).

The connection between personality and friendship remains to be explored. A next step in terms of research in this area would be to investigate how identity, generativity, and confident power affects women's friendships at midlife. One prediction might be that women's established friendships will gain in importance and clarity at midlife for those women who become self-actualized. It may also be the case that establishing friendships may become more difficult or less eagerly approached at midlife. Paul (2004) explained that, by midlife, one is more aware of what effort is involved in starting a friendship:

> The chocolate cake in the cooking magazine immediately snared me. The triple layers of dark devil's food—my favorite—were glazed with a rich, fudgy ganache. I'd been craving chocolate cake. I could almost taste it. Maybe I'd share it with my family, maybe not. Then I noticed the length list of ingredients, including an artisan chocolate that had to be specially ordered from a catalog. The recipe was complicated – carefully melting chocolate in a double boiler and whipping egg whites. Way too much trouble. Even though I knew it would be delicious, I turned the page. New friendships can feel like that. (p. 90)

Cross-cultural Perspectives

People in numerous cultures characterize the friendship process as one of increasing levels of intimacy. Despite the universality of the process, the character of friendship varies cross-culturally. Some rules of friendship appear to cut across culture; other rules suggest that differences in cultural values might affect friendship. Argyle and Henderson (1984) reported that adults from Britain, Hong Kong, Japan, and Italy (ages 18 to 25 and 30 to 60) endorsed four common rules of friendship: respect the other's privacy, trust and confide in one another, volunteer help in time of need, and avoid jealousy or criticism of the friend's relationships. However, Japanese adults gave more weight than the other three groups did to the friend fulfilling ritual obligations, providing help if requested, and offering information and regard, and they gave less weight than the other groups did to verbal intimacy and supportiveness.

The dimension of individualism–collectivism has been used to explain many differences in interpersonal behaviors, including friendship. The difference between the Japanese and the other cultures above may be attributable to the individualism–collectivism dimension; perhaps intimacy is more highly regarded in individualistic (Western) societies and fulfillment of formal obligations is more important in collectivist (Eastern) societies.

If we extrapolate from that study, we might hypothesize that women in collectivist societies would have more close friends than women in individualist societies. An alternative hypothesis is that women in collectivist cultures would have fewer but closer friends than do women in individualist cultures. The latter hypothesis was partially borne out by a study of adults from West Africa (Ghana) and North America (Adams & Plaut, 2003), although gender effects were not reported separately. West Africans had fewer friends than North Americans, and the friendship expectations of the two groups also differed. Significantly more West Africans expected material and practical support and guidance, correction, and warning, whereas more North Americans expected emotional support, trust, and respect. Thus, a limited amount of cross-cultural research suggests that gender and culture both are significant factors in determining friendship patterns between women from other cultures.

Conflict, False Friends, and Bad Friends

"Are Friends Delight or Pain?" asked Emily Dickinson (Enright & Rawlinson, 1991, p. 317). Friends are a major source of conflict as well as rewards. Conflict is likely to arise when the rules of friendship are broken. The most important rules to keep in friendship, according to adults from four cultures, are as follows: share news of success with each other; show emotional support; volunteer help in time of need; and strive to make the friend happy when in each other's company (Argyle & Furnham, 1983). Conflict in friendship also could result from one partner's reliance on exchange norms rather than communal norms (Clark, 1981). If one friend persists in basing the friendship on an explicitly even exchange, such as expecting every phone call or invitation to be returned before another is extended, the friendship may be damaged. Established friendships tend to operate based on communal norms, such that friends expect to give according to abilities and needs rather than according to a strict system of even exchange. Thus, the expectation might be that the friend with more free time would be the one to take the lead in organizing get-togethers, whereas the busy friend would contribute to the friendship in some other way.

Responses to Conflict

Responses to conflict may determine friendship outcomes. Four types of responses to conflict have been identified: exit, voice, loyalty, and neglect (Rusbult et al., 1982). Exit responses refer to threatening to end the friendship, discussing ending it, driving the friend away, or actually ending the friendship. *Voice* includes responses such as talking about the problem, recommending solutions, compromising, or trying to change the friend or the self. *Loyalty* responses refer to waiting to see if things improve or continuing to have faith in the friendship or the self. Last, *neglect* responses refer to ignoring the friend, spending less time together, refusing to talk about the problem, or complaining without suggesting solutions.

Typically, friends tend to adopt passive responses to conflict in friendship, such as loyally continuing the friendships despite dissatisfaction or by neglecting the friend (e.g., Fehr & Harasymchuk, 2005). Because passive responses are the norm, active responses to conflict, such as threatening to end the friendship or voicing the issue, might be regarded as disruptions in the usual way of dealing with things. People expect friendships to be "self-maintaining" and thus, a friend who responds to conflict more actively may be a surprise. On the other hand, a friendship could be strengthened by a friend's attentive response to an expression of dissatisfaction.

The research on conflict raises at least two questions concerning mature women's friendships that have yet to be addressed. First, are older women quicker to react to conflict in friendship or more active in resolving it than young women are? Predictions vary. It could be that older women would be more patient in waiting for conflicts to resolve spontaneously. In contrast, if the friendship is not rewarding, they may be more willing than young women to end it. Second, are older women better at predicting a friend's response or selecting the most successful way to handle the conflict with that particular friend? It might be expected that older women, who have sustained long-term friendships, have developed ways to cope with problems successfully. A stable interpersonal script based on long intimacy may govern friendships; a woman may know what friends respond to neglect and what friends appreciate an active approach to problems. In other words, older women's life experience and in-depth knowledge of friends might broaden their repertoire concerning how to handle conflicts.

False Friends and Bad Friends

Research has shown that people with strong friendships experience less stress, recover more quickly from heart attacks, and are likely to live longer than the friendless. They are even more resistant to the common cold (Pressman et al., 2005). Further, more positive health outcomes occur for individuals when they affiliate with a friend in response to a stressful situation; women have a greater tendency than men do to "tend and befriend" when under stress (Taylor et al., 2000). However, some friends may do more harm than good. The extent to which friendships might be destructive or bad for one's health is just beginning to be explored (Yager, 2002). In an enduring friendship, as in any deep relationship, anger, jealousy, envy, and other difficult emotions may occur. Also, some friends lie, cling, criticize, or betray. One may have to decide whether it is just a phase in the friendship and ride it out, or whether it is a permanent condition and disband it.

Betrayal in friendship may be particularly hurtful. Violating a confidence is regarded as a serious affront to a friendship, and Yager (2002) identified 20 additional different types of bad friends. The second most harmful type is when a friend suddenly turns cold without explaining why. This is perceived as more than just an abandonment; the silent treatment is malicious. A third type of bad friend involves someone who insults the other person. The most common type is the promise breaker, someone who promises to be there when needed, then isn't. Some friendships go bad when one of the people gradually or suddenly finds reasons to dislike the other one. It sometimes may take a long while in a friendship to learn enough about the friend to violate one's "dislike criteria," that is, to discover that the friend is a liar, not to be trusted, or that the costs of the friendship greatly outweigh the rewards.

In sum, good friendships are known to contribute to psychological health, but it is becoming apparent that false and bad friendships create stress and do harm. What remains to be explored is if women at midlife are more likely than younger or older women to break off from stressful or harmful friendships.

Directions for Research

Clearly, a great deal about women's friendships has yet to be explained. There are many potential directions for future research. Merely extending any major area of friendship research to include women at midlife would be a good start. For instance, research on expectations, intimacy, communication, conflict, maintenance, or gender differences in any of these areas targeted at women in midlife would begin to build a profile of adult women's friendships. Studies of the strategies women use to establish and maintain friendships and the processes of transition from one phase of friendship to another are particularly lacking (Bleiszner & Roberto, 2004). In addition, little is known about the importance of friends in accomplishing generative goals such as volunteering to help develop community programs or providing opportunities for mentorship (Antonnuci & Akiyama, 1997).

Longitudinal studies using a narrative analysis also might provide a rich context for exploring the convergence of social cognition, life stage, and friendship development. Narratives refer to the stories people create and recreate that help them to interpret and explain relationships. They are important because they help people make sense of their lives (Knapp & Miller, 1994). Many women have long-term and even lifelong friendships that could be tracked over time using narratives or stories about those friendships to examine how identity and cognitions interact with friendship processes and meanings.

Yet another unique approach would be to use women's midlife friendships as a normative model for the study of other relationships and processes. This would be a novel undertaking, particularly because women's friendships traditionally have been regarded as secondary to marital, parental, family, and work relationships. Yet a great deal of research in those areas is aimed at how to avoid problems or how to make those relationships more effective. One could argue that because women's midlife friendships seem to be somewhat protected from the level of disappointment and conflict experienced in romantic and marital relationships, they might provide some insight as to the conditions required to make marriage more positive and fulfilling. In other words, a good friendship might be the best basis for many types of relationships, and women's midlife friendships might serve as an example of how to have them.

The Future of Women's Friendship

The immediate future of women's friendships after age 50 will be affected by the intersection of four forces: lifespan development, life course transitions, caring experiences over the life course, and the sociohistorical context (Bleiszner, 2006). The lifespan development perspective suggests that a key challenge throughout life is to adapt to developmental gains and losses, such as children leaving home, widowhood, or divorce. For example, although loneliness and loss may accompany widowhood, it also provides opportunities for developing other interests and friendships (Adams, 1987). Life transitions also play a role in women's friendships after 50. The impact of life transitions is determined by the age at which they occur. Women in their 50s who are caring for aging parents may have more constraints on their friendships than their age peers who are not; whereas the death of a parent may increase a woman's reliance on her friends. Caring refers to feeling and exhibiting concern and empathy for others. Lifespan perspectives suggest that women who have positive experiences with caring in early and middle adulthood will be more likely to have caring and intimate friendships in the later years of life. Current sociohistorical influences also are expected to play a role in women's friendships. For example, members of the baby boom cohort are likely to view friendships differently in old age than the previous generation did. The prediction is that baby boomers will have mainly age-homogeneous friendships because of to the strong cohort identity they forged in their youth due to sharing powerful historical events together such as the Vietnam War (Bleiszner, 2006).

The beginning of the twenty-first century has been marked by tremendous changes that will continue to affect friendships (Allan, 2001). The introduction of mass-scale, worldwide, electronic communication and continuing globalization has had an impact on women's everyday lives and relationships. More women work outside the home, and in industrialized nations women may expect to live for nearly a century. Marriage has become less normative, and divorce quite soon may be the majority pattern. Overall, women are having fewer children and their dependency on men is declining. As a result, "the domestic, sexual, and familial arrangements that adults construct are now perceived far more as a personal matter for those involved and not as issues over which others have strong rights to influence" (Allan, 2001, p. 329).

These changes have large implications for informal relationships like friendship. Friendship is likely to become an even more important part of social identity as women become freer to develop nondomestic aspects of their lives. Friendship may also play an increasingly important role in confirming new decisions or changes that are made. Lesbian identities provide a good example. Friendships are highly significant for many lesbians for whom friends represent their "chosen family" (Weeks et al., 2001). These are the friends who are trusted and relied upon. Widowed and divorced heterosexual women as they age potentially might begin to adopt a similar model of establishing a "chosen family" comprised of friends.

Signs that women after 50 will forge new directions for friendship already have begun to appear. The Red Hat Society, which has chapters in dozens of cities, is an example of women using friendship ties to promote a more positive cultural view of women after age 50. Red Hat Society members wear red hats and purple clothing to symbolize that after age 50 women will make their own choices about what is fashionable. As founder Sue Ellen Cooper explained:

"The Red Hat Society began as a result of a few women deciding to greet middle age with verve, humor and elan. We believe silliness is the comedy relief of life, and since we are all in it together, we might as well join red-gloved hands and go for the gusto together. Underneath the frivolity, we share a bond of affection, forged by common life experiences and a genuine enthusiasm for wherever life takes us next." (http://www.redhatsociety.com)

The establishment of intentional or retirement communities organized by groups of women friends might also arise after age 50 in response to the declining sex ratio of men to women in the later decades of life. Communities based on lesbian friendships and networks already have been established in Florida, Arizona, and

Washington (Rabin & Slater, 2005). The Florida location was founded in 1995 and currently has 330 residents on 278 landscaped home sites within 50 acres of gated, fenced land (Rabin & Slater, 2005). The model of the lesbian residential/retirement community might become a viable type of community structure for heterosexual women friends in the future, as well.

The feminist potential of women's friendships in the future remains to be seen. Irigaray (1985) argued that interaction between women enables them to define a self that transcends the limits imposed on women by patriarchal language and culture. Interactions between women may not always be harmonious, but they allow women a new and different way of being that cannot appear when women are defined by the needs, desires, and fantasies of men. If women's friendships become more significant as they age, they have the potential to challenge the centrality of men in women's lives. This could lead women to recognize and use their power in the public arena. The functions of women's friendships could broaden beyond intimacy and ego support to include instrumental ones, such as access to economic and political resources, much as men's friendships do (O'Connor, 1998). Thus, women's friendships after 50 potentially have important implications for feminist and political activism. Guttentag and Secord (1983) theorized that feminist movements tend to develop when women greatly outnumber men. If so, in the future, women over 50 may become an important base of political influence and social change.

In conclusion, it remains to be seen if women's friendships will continue to reinforce women's place in the private sphere, as defined by patriarchy, or will become a catalyst for their entry into the public arena. However, current trends suggest that friendship in the future will become increasingly important across the lifespan, particularly so among women after age 50 who will have the greatest opportunity to construct their own place in the world.

References

Adams, R.G. (1997). Friendship patterns among older women. In J.M. Coyle (Ed.), *Handbook on Women and Aging* (pp. 400–417). Westport, CT: Greenwood.

Adams, G., and Plaut, V.C. (2003). The cultural grounding of personal relationship: Friendships in North American and West African worlds. *Personal Relationships, 10*, 333–347.

Allan, G. (1998). Friendships and the private sphere. In R.G. Adams and G. Allan (Eds.), *Placing Friendship in Context* (pp. 92–116). Cambridge: Cambridge University Press.

Allan, G. (2001). Personal relationships in late modernity. *Personal Relationships, 8*, 325–339.

Antonucci, T., and Akiyama, H. (1997). Concern with others at midlife: Care, comfort, or compromise? In M.E. Lachman and J.B. James (Eds.), *Multiple Paths of Midlife Development* (pp. 147–169). Chicago: University of Chicago Press.

Argyle, M., and Furnham, A. (1983). Sources of satisfaction and conflict in long-term relationships. *Journal of Marriage and the Family, 45*, 481–493.

Argyle, M., and Henderson, M. (1984). The rules of friendship. *Journal of Social and Personal Relationships, 1*, 211–238.

Armstrong, M.J., and Goldsteen, K.S. (1990). Friendship support patterns of older American women. *Journal of Aging Studies, 4*, 391–404.

Bank, B.J. (1995). Friendships in Australia and the United States: From feminization to a more heroic image. *Gender & Society, 9*, 79–98.

Bank, B.J., and Hansford, S.L. (2003). Gender and friendship: Why are men's best same-sex friendships less intimate and supportive? *Personal Relationships, 7*, 63–78.

Basow, S.A., and Rubenfeld, K. (2003). "Troubles talk": Effects of gender and gender typing. *Sex Roles, 48*, 183–187.

Bell, S., and Coleman, S. (Eds.). (1999). *The Anthropology of Friendship.* Oxford: Berg.

Bleiszner, R. (2006). A lifetime of caring: Dimensions and dynamics in late-life close relationships. *Personal Relationships, 13*, 1–18.

Bleiszner, R., and Adams, R.G. (1992). *Adult Friendship.* Newbury Park, CA: Sage.

Bleiszner, R., and Roberto, K.A. (2004). Friendship across the life span: Reciprocity in individual and relationship development. In F.R. Lang and K.L. Fingerman (Eds.), *Growing Together: Personal Relationships Across the Lifespan* (pp. 159–182). Cambridge: Cambridge University Press.

Bradford, J., and Ryan, C. (1991). Who we are: Health concerns of middle-aged lesbians. In B. Sang, J. Warshow, and A. Smith (Eds.), *Lesbians at Midlife: The Creative Transition* (pp.147–163). San Francisco: Spinsters Ink.

Cartwright, L.K., and Wink, P. (1994). Personality change in women physicians from medical student years to mid-40s. *Psychology of Women Quarterly,* 18, 291–308.

Clark, M.S. (1981). Noncomparability of benefits given and received: A cue to the existence of friendship. *Social Psychology Quarterly, 44*, 375–381.

Clark, M.S., and Mills, J. (1993). The difference between communal and exchange relationships: What it is and is not. *Personality and Social Psychology Bulletin, 19*, 684–691.

Enright, D.J., and Rawlinson, D. (1992). *The Oxford Book of Friendship.* New York: Oxford University Press.

Erikson, E.H. (1968). *Identity: Youth and Crisis.* New York: Norton.

Faderman, L. (1981). *Surpassing the Love of Men.* New York: Morrow.

Fehr, B. (1996). *Friendship Processes.* Thousand Oaks, CA: Sage.

Fehr, B., and Harasymchuk, C. (2005). The experience of emotion in close relationships: Toward an integration of the emotion-in-relationships and interpersonal script models. *Personal Relationships, 12*, 181–196.

Gersick, C.J., and Kram, K.E. (2002). High achieving women at midlife: An exploratory study. *Journal of Management Inquiry, 11*, 104–127.

Goodenow, C., and Gaier, E.L. (1990, August). *Best Friends: The Close Reciprocal Friendships of Married and Unmarried Women.* Paper presented at the meeting of the American Psychological Association, Washington, DC.

Gouldner, H., and Strong, M.S. (1987). *Speaking of Friendship: Middle-class Women and Their Friends.* Westport, CT: Greenwood.

Green, E., Hebron, S., and Woodward, D. (1990). *Women's Leisure: What Leisure?* Basingstoke, UK: Macmillan.

Greenberg, S., and Motenko, A.K. (1994). Women growing older: Partnerships for change. In M.P. Mirkin (Ed.), *Women in Context: Toward a Feminist Reconstruction of Psychotherapy* (pp. 96–117). New York: Guilford.

Gullestad, M. (1984). *Kitchen Table Society.* Oslo: Universities Forlaget.

Guttentag, M., and Secord, P. (1983). *Too Many Women? The Sex Ratio Question.* Beverly Hills, CA: Sage.

Hall, R., and Rose, S. (1996). Friendships between African-American and White lesbians. In J.S. Weinstock and E.D. Rothblum (Eds.), *Lesbian Friendships: For Ourselves and Each Other* (pp. 165–191). New York: New York University Press.

Holmstrom, A.J., Burleson, B.R., and Jones, S.M. (2005). Some consequences for helpers who deliver "cold comfort": Why it's worse for women than men to be inept when providing emotional support. *Sex Roles, 53*, 153–172.

Irigaray, L. (1985). *This Sex Which Is Not One*. New York: Cornell University Press.

Keefe, S.E., Padilla, A.M., and Carlos, M.L. (1979). The Mexican-American extended family as an emotional support system. *Human Organization, 38*, 144–152.

Kimmel, D.C., and Sang, B.E. (1995). Lesbians and gay men in midlife. In A.R. D'Augelli and C.J. Patterson (Eds.), *Lesbian, Gay, and Bisexual Identities Over the Lifespan: Psychological Perspectives* (pp. 190–214). New York: Oxford University Press.

Kitzinger, C. (1996). Toward a politics of lesbian friendship. In J.S. Weinstock and E.D. Rothblum (Eds.), *Lesbian friendships: For ourselves and each other* (pp. 295–299). New York: New York University Press.

Knapp, M.R., and Miller, G.R. (1994). *Handbook of Interpersonal Communication* (2nd ed.). Thousand Oaks, CA: Sage.

Krause, N., and Borawski-Clark, E. (Eds.) (1995). Social class differences in social support among older adults. *Gerontologist, 35*, 498–508.

Larson, R.W., and Bradney, N. (1988). Precious moments with family members and friends. In R.W. Larson, N. Bradney, and R.M. Milardo (Eds.), *Families and Social Networks. New Perspectives on Family* (pp. 107–126). Thousand Oaks, CA: Sage.

Levine, S.B. (2005). *Inventing the Rest of Our Lives: Women in Second Adulthood*. London: Viking Press.

Lewittes, H.J. (1989). Just being friendly means a lot–Women, friendship, and aging. In L. Grace and I. Susser (Eds.), *Women in the Later Years: Health, Social, and Cultural Perspectives* (pp. 138–159). New York: Harrington Park Press.

Masheter, C. (1997). Healthy and unhealthy friendship and hostility between ex-spouses. *Journal of Marriage and the Family, 59*, 207–222.

Nardi, P.M., and Sherrod, D. (1994). Friendships in the lives of gay men and lesbians. *Journal of Social and Personal Relationships, 11*, 185–199.

Neugarten, B.L. (1968). The awareness of middle age. In B.L. Neugarten (Ed.), *Middle Age and Aging* (pp. 93–98). Chicago: University of Chicago Press.

O'Connor, P. (1992). *Friendships between Women*. New York: Guilford.

O'Connor, P. (1998). Women's friendships in a post-modern world. In R.G. Adams and G. Allan (Eds.), *Placing friendship in context* (pp. 117–135). Cambridge: Cambridge University Press.

Patrick, J.H., Cottrell, L.E., and Barnes, K.A. (2001). Gender, emotional support, and well-being among the rural elderly. *Sex Roles, 45*, 15–29.

Paul, M. (2004). *The Friendship Crisis: Finding, Making, and Keeping Friends When You're Not a Kid Anymore*. Emmaus, PA: Rodale.

Pressman, S.D., Cohen, S., Miller, G.E., Barkin, A., Rabin, B.S., and Treanor, J.J. (2005). Loneliness, social network size, and immune response to influenza vaccination in college freshmen. *Health Psychology, 24*, 297–306.

Rabin, J., and Slater, B.R. (2005). Lesbian communities across the United States: Pockets of resistance and resilience. *Journal of Lesbian Studies, 9*, 169–182.

Rodriguez, N., Mira, C.B., Myers, H.F., Morris, J.K., and Cardoza, D. (2003). Family or friends: Who plays a greater supportive role for Latino college students? *Cultural Diversity and Ethnic Minority Psychology, 9*, 236–250.

Roberto, K.A. (2001). Older women's relationships: Weaving lives together. In J.D. Garner and S.O. Mercer (Eds.), *Women as They Age* (2nd ed., pp. 115–129). New York: Haworth.

Rose, S.M. (1984). How friendships end. *Journal of Social and Personal Relationships, 1,* 267–278.

Rose, S. (2000). Heterosexism and the study of women's romantic and friend relationships. *Journal of Social Issues, 56,* 315–328.

Rothblum, E.D., Mintz, B., Cowan, D.B., and Haller, C. (1995). Lesbian baby boomers at midlife. In K. Jay (Ed.), *Dyke Life: From Growing Up to Growing Old-A celebration of the Lesbian Experience* (pp. 61–76). New York: Basic Books.

Rusbult, C.E., Zembrodt, I.M., and Gunn, L.K. (1982). Exit, voice, loyalty, and neglect: Responses to dissatisfaction in romantic involvements. *Journal of Personality and Social Psychology, 43,* 1230–1242.

Samter, W., Whaley, B.B., Mortenson, S.T., and Burleson, B.R. (1997). Ethnicity and emotional support in same-sex friendship: A comparison of Asian-Americans, African-Americans, and Euro-Americans. *Personal Relationships, 4,* 413–430.

Sang, B. (1991). Moving toward balance and integration. In B. Sang, J. Warshow, and A. Smith (Eds.), *Lesbians at Midlife: The Creative Transition* (pp. 206–214). San Francisco: Spinsters Ink.

Stanley, J.L. (1996). The lesbian's experience of friendship. In J.S. Weinstock and E.D. Rothblum (Eds.), *Lesbian Friendships: For Ourselves and Each Other* (pp. 39–59). New York: New York University Press.

Stewart, A.J., Ostrove, J.M., and Helson, R. (2001). Middle aging in women: Patterns of personality change from the 30s to 50s. *Journal of Adult Development, 8,* 23–27.

Tangri, S.S., Thomas, V.G., Mednick, M.T., and Lee, K.S. (2003). Predictors of satisfaction among college-educated Black women in midlife. *Journal of Adult Development, 10,* 113–135.

Taylor, S.E., Klein, L.C., Lewis, B.P., Gruenewald, T.L., Gurung, R.A., and Updegraff, R., (2000). Biobehavioral responses to stress in females: Tend-and-befriend, not fight-or-flight. *Psychological Review, 107,* 411–429.

Trotman, F.K., and Brody, C.M. (Eds.) (2002). *Psychotherapy and Counseling with Older Women*. New York: Springer.

Tully, C.T. (1989). Domestic violence: The ultimate betrayal of human rights. *Journal of Lesbian and Gay Social Services, 13,* 83–98.

Vandeventer, E.A., Ostrove, J.M., and Stewart, A.J. (1997). Predicting women's well-being in midlife: The importance of personality development and social role involvement. *Journal of Personality and Social Psychology, 72,* 1147–1160.

Weeks, J., Heaphy, B., and Donovan, C. (2001). *Same Sex Intimacies: Families of Choice and Other Life Experiments*. New York: Routledge.

Weinstock, J.S. (2000). Lesbian, gay, bisexual and transgender friendships in adulthood: Review and analysis. In C.J. Patterson and A.R. D'Augelli (Eds.), *Lesbian, Gay, and Bisexual Identities in Families: Psychological Perspectives* (pp. 122–153). New York: Oxford University Press.

Weinstock, J.S. (2004). Lesbian flexibility: Friend and/or family connections among lesbian ex-lovers. *Journal of Lesbian Studies, 8,* 193–238.

Weston, K. (1997). *Families we choose: Lesbians, gays, kinship* (rev. ed.). New York: Columbia University Press. [Originally published 1991.]

Yager, J. (2002). *When Friendship Hurts: How to Deal with Friends Who Betray, Abandon, or Wound You*. New York: Fireside.

7
Contemporary Midlife Grandparenthood

Liat Kulik

Grandparenthood has always been considered a basic human experience, and usually it is a positive one. The grandparent role is salient for most older individuals (Cherlin & Furstenberg, 1985), and some scholars have argued that its impact on the individual and family will continue to grow (Uhlenberg & Kirby, 1998). Today, grandparenting can span several decades, from the 30s in cases of teenage pregnancy, to over 100 years of age in cases of extreme longevity (Hagestad, 1985). Although it is difficult to determine whether the grandparent role is more significant than the roles of spouse and parent, there is no doubt that becoming a grandparent is a milestone in the life cycle, and, as such, it is of considerable relevance to self-identity. From a developmental perspective, because the transition to grandparenthood symbolizes a new stage of life, it is an especially important component of age identity (Bastida, 1987; Giarrusso et al., 1996). From a psychosocial perspective, the experience of grandparenting is influenced by synchronicity with other events in the older person's life (Troll, 1985). Accordingly, a person's behavior in the grandparent role and the significance attributed to grandparenting are influenced by other major life cycle events, such as changes in marital and work status.

The grandparent role has been defined as a "roleless role," or a role that is not governed by rights and obligations to the same extent as the parent role (Clavan, 1978). Based on a combination of perspectives presented in the literature, Kahana and Kahana (1971) proposed a complex conceptualization of grandparenthood. According to this conceptualization, grandparenthood is a social role that involves ascribed status and expectations for role performance vis-à-vis the family and the society. Grandparenthood also can be viewed as an emotional state or an intrapsychic experience, which is part of individual development (Kornhaber & Woodward, 1981). In that context, grandparenthood is a transaction between the grandchild and grandparent, which involves reciprocity (Werner, 1991). Grandparenthood can also be viewed as part a group process within the family, which involves relationships and interdependencies among three generations (Cohler & Gruenbaum, 1981). Finally, grandparenthood can be considered a symbol. It is a reflection of continuity, potency, and usefulness to society (Troll, 1983; Werner, 1991). From any point of view, it is clear that far-reaching changes in modern society are also reflected in the grandparent role.

In line with the developmental and psychosocial approaches described above, the significance attributed to the grandparent role and styles of grandparenting are usually affected by the sociocultural environment and by the stage of life in which the event occurs. In this chapter, I will attempt to shed light on the significance of grandparenthood in the contemporary period, with emphasis on an aspect that has been neglected in existing research, namely grandmothers in their 50s.

Grandparenting in a Rapidly Changing Environment

The social, ideological, technological, and political developments of the contemporary era are reflected in every sphere of life. These developments have affected the roles that individuals fulfill in the family, including grandparenting. Regarding the changes that have affected the experience of grandparenting, several areas are noteworthy.

Increased Life Expectancy

Advancements in medical technology and increased emphasis on healthy life styles have led to a significant rise in life expectancy in Western countries. Whereas very few children had living grandparents at the turn of the previous century, today this is no longer the case. Ninety percent of all North American children at age 10 and 75% of all children at age 20 have at least one living grandparent. At the same time, most older people have grandchildren. In the late 1970s, about 75% of all older adults had experienced grandparenthood (Barranti, 1985; Hagestad, 1985), and today some older people are even great–great grandparents. According to Canadian researchers, 75% to 80% of older Canadians have at least one grandchild, and the majority have more. In the United States, over 90% of all older people with children also have grandchildren (for a review, see Schlesinger & Schlesinger, 1998). As a result of increased longevity, many people will be grandparents for one-half of their lifetime (Barranti, 1985), over a period that can last as long as 30 years. However, owing to a decline in fertility rates, there will be fewer grandchildren per family—although the grandparent–grandchild relationship will last longer and may be more intensive. Thus, grandparents can potentially have a stronger influence on each one of their grandchildren than in the past.

Multiple and Simultaneous Family Roles

As a result of increased longevity, a person can also fulfill multiple roles at a given point in life, for example, it is possible simultaneously to be a parent, grandparent, great grandparent, and even a great–great grandparent in extreme cases. In Israel, among Yemenite Jews who marry at a young age and often live to be very old, there are five-generation families in which the great–great grandparent is known as a *hamis*. Not only can one individual perform several family roles at the same time, but each role is characterized by diverse characteristics and patterns. Several decades ago, for example, the age range of children in a family tended to be relatively homogeneous. Today, at the same point in time one person can be a parent to married offspring, and still have adolescents or even infants living at home. This creates complex situations, in which one person needs to use a variety of parenting skills in order to satisfy the needs of children who are at different stages of life. There are situations, albeit not common ones, in which a person can have grandchildren and offspring of the same age, or even offspring who are younger than the grandchildren. There are several reasons for the prolonged period of parenthood and diverse age range of children. First, in light of increased rates of divorce and remarriage, the remarried couple may wish to have children of their own, in addition to the children that each spouse has from a previous marriage. Furthermore, especially with the advancements in medical technology, there is an increasing tendency for women to give birth in middle age and prolong the fertility period. Thus, when a woman reaches an age where she is about to become a grandmother, she may conceive one last child of her own out of a desire to prove her femininity, to cement a new marriage, or to prolong motherhood to the maximum. In Israel, the tendency to give birth in middle age (and even at the age of grandparenthood) is particularly significant among ultra-Orthodox Jewish women, who view procreation as a divine commandment and seek to have as many children as possible during the period of fertility. Furthermore, in light of persistent military tension in Israeli society, there are couples who lose a son or daughter in war or in a terrorist attack. In these cases, the couple might conceive a child at a relatively late stage of life in order to fill the vacuum and in an attempt to rehabilitate the family.

Diversity in the nature of family roles may also derive from changes in family structure as a result of divorce and separation, remarriage, and blending of families. Thus, at one and the same time, a grandparent can have biological and step-grandchildren. For example, in cases of midlife remarriage, a person can act as a step-parent to the new spouse's children and as a step-grandparent to that spouse's grandchildren. Moreover, when divorced offspring remarry, a grandparent can acquire step-children (the new spouse of their offspring) as well as step-grandchildren. These multiple and diverse family roles can be a source of pleasure to some individuals in the modern world (including grandparents), but can also generate stress and confusion of self-identity.

Increased Diversity of the Family Configuration

One of the characteristics of the family in postmodern society is the diversity of the family configuration. Different configurations include single-parent families (sometimes out of choice, and not necessarily as a result of separation or divorce), "blended" families (the husband's children from a former marriage, the wife's children from a former marriage, and the children they have together), lesbian or gay families, and cohabiting families. In addition, there are families in which earning patterns and division of labor differ from the traditional ones known in the past. For example, there are dual-career families, in which both spouses focus on developing their careers, but one spouse bears the main responsibility for maintaining the household. In some cases, both spouses earn about the same income ("modern" families), and in other cases the wife is the main provider and the husband sometimes cares for the household ("innovators") (Izraeli, 1994). Even though these configurations include families that are not distressed or at risk, and even families that are relatively well-off, there are families that experience a certain degree of instability due to the excessive burden on one or both parents and due to ambiguous gender roles or parental roles. In these situations, grandparents are often called on to lend a hand and to help maintain stability in the family (Kornhaber, 1996).

The Diverse Functions of Grandparenthood

Grandmothers have always played a supportive role in the family (Robertson, 1977). They are believed to engage voluntarily in bargaining and exchange with grandchildren, or offer help with educational expenses (Sussman, 1953, 1962). However, the role of grandparents in contemporary society has expanded and intensified due to social changes that have weakened the family unit, increased pressures on families, and increased rates of children at risk. Thus, grandparents (especially grandmothers) are called on increasingly by their families and society to help their children and grandchildren (Kornhaber, 1996). Households headed by grandparents are clearly on the rise due to teenage pregnancy, incompetent parenting, child abuse, divorce, and illness (Burton, 1992; Creighton, 1991; Minkler & Roe, 1993).

Other recent social phenomena that have had a major impact on the grandparent role are drug addition, AIDS, and incarceration (Burton, 1992; Dressel & Barnhill, 1994; Minkler & Roe, 1993). In such cases, grandparents play a primary role as surrogate parents to their grandchildren. Regarding incarceration, the rates of women in prison have increased by 20% over the past decade (Dressel & Barnhill, 1994), and approximately 53% of the children of incarcerated mothers live with their grandparents (Bahr, 1994). In addition, grandmothers can be called on to help with grandchildren who have chronic difficulties (e.g., developmental disabilities, physical illnesses). In those cases, the grandparents serve as stress buffers, and make an important contribution to countering negative forces in their children's lives (Denham & Smith, 1989). Thus, grandparents can often act as babysitters (Lajewski, 1959) or surrogate parents (Kornhaber, 1996), and can intervene at times of crisis and disaster (Young, 1959). At the same time, they can act as bearers of family history and tradition (Boyd, 1967), and they can help in the household when parents are ill, giving birth, or on vacation (Sussman, 1962), as well as supplement the family income by giving gifts. In a somewhat different vein, grandparents can also act as companions and confidants to their grandchildren, in addition to mitigating tension in families (Neugarten & Weinstein, 1964).

Breaking the Stereotype of the Traditional Grandparent—Diversity of Styles

In the not so distant past, the grandmother's role was fairly standard and clearly defined. "Grandma" was considered a relatively uniform, homogeneous figure, and was portrayed in the media and in children's literature as a woman who does not work for pay. Whether she had never held a job or whether she was retired, her main role was to manage the home and help to take care of her grandchildren. In a similar vein, the stereotype of the old grandmother has prevailed for years (Smith, 1995). A study (Jannelli, 1988) conducted among North American children between 1961 and 1983 revealed 55% of the participants portrayed grandmothers as having white or graying hair, 31% portrayed them as wearing glasses, and 31% portrayed them as wearing aprons. Researchers who have attempted to identify different styles of grandmothering have usually focused on one main dimension, that is, grandmother–grandchildren relationships (Deutsch, 1945; Robertson, 1976). In this connection, Neugarten and Weinstein (1964) formulated a classic typology of grandmotherhood, which identified grandmothering styles along a continuum of grandparent–grandchild relations, and revealed the following main types: *the formal type* reflects the grandparents who do what they are "supposed to do"; the *fun seekers* are grandparents who play with their grandchildren, and they are usually relatively young; *surrogate grandparents* are those who take care of their grandchildren while the parents are away; the *reservoir of family wisdom* refers to grandparents who are authoritative figures and teach special skills; and the *distant figure* is the grandparent who is benevolent but remote.

Today, the images of grandmothers and styles of grandmotherhood are diverse, as reflected in the media where one grandmother wears a jogging suit on her way to aerobic dancing, and another wears a business suit and has a successful career (Hagestad, 1985). In Israel, there is a popular children's book entitled *Grandma in Jeans* (Orbach, 2001), which portrays a grandmother who is young at heart—an image completely the opposite of the classic grandmother stereotype. Hence, the images of grandmothers are more varied than ever before, and there is increasing social legitimacy for every grandmother to choose the image that best suits her.

Breaking the Myth of the "Happy Grandmother"

Another stereotype about grandmothers that prevailed in the past is that grandmotherhood is an entirely happy experience. In many studies (e.g., Timberlake, 1986), grandparents have described their relationship with their grandchildren as fulfilling. They portray their role in a positive light, as a source of stability, continuity, care, consistency, and routine to their grandchildren. From that perspective, Johnson (1983) presented two descriptions of the grandparenting experience: "It's a deeper love than between a parent and child, because it is coming from a loved one (a child) and a result of loving and being loved" (p. 554); "being a grandparent has all the good points—'have them [the grandchildren] over when you choose, and send them home when they act bratty'" (p. 553). Some have described grandparenthood as bliss: "Being Daphna's grandmother is the ultimate bliss, the crème de la crème. When little Daphna opens the door shouts 'grandma, grandma,' I am filled to the brim with happiness, and there's no other feeling like it" (Kulik, 2005).

Today, it seems that these feelings are accompanied by other voices, which shatter the prevailing image of grandparenthood as the ultimate happiness. These voices reflect changes in the women's perceptions of self-fulfillment, as well as changing aspirations, and portray a more balanced view of being a grandmother. According to Johnson (1983), some women described a conflict between their role as a grandmother, and emphasized other interests and aspirations in life: "I am just not the grandmother type—I travel, take courses, have my own interests... I have my own life to lead, and so do my grandchildren" (p. 554). In a similar vein, Goodfellow (2003) cited the following response: "My friend had trouble with her young grandchild, who would not want to go home because he had been with her 12 hours and more a day" (p. 5). Another response to the experience of grandmotherhood is the fear of growing old, as reflected in the following statements: "I'm too young to be a grandmother" (Johnson, 1983, p. 554); "If I had enough guts, I would tell my children to wait a while before they start a family. Grandchildren will bring me into another stage of life, and I feel like I'm still a child myself" (Kulik, 2005). Some grandmothers complain about feeling bored when they are with their grandchildren: "I get bored sitting and playing with her [the grandchild] and doing things like drawing and playing with playdough" (Goodfellow, 2003, p. 6). Sometimes the transition to grandmotherhood in midlife forces women to confront the fact that they will not bear any more children and that the childbearing function will be passed on to the next generation. As one grandmother expressed it: "When my first grandchild was born, I felt that a biological stage of my life had ended, the stage of childbearing... but in a strange way I returned to my own experience of childbearing and child rearing. I was filled with memories from that time, nostalgia... It was the most beautiful period of my life—and now, with the birth of my grandchild, I realize how I can't turn the wheels back..." (Kulik, 2005). The transition to grandmotherhood can also generate inner conflict, for example, when the new grandmother thinks that her children are taking advantage of her, as described by Goodfellow (2003): "I used to have my grandson for breakfast, give him his meals, bathe him at night, and get him ready for bed... so what does his mother do?" (p. 6).

Goodfellow (2003) also described strain caused by the overload that ensues when the grandmother feels drained by the responsibility of taking care of grandchildren: "I sometimes feel tied down. It's really hard to look after your grandchild, particularly when the child's parents want to go out (socially) or I have something I want to do" (p. 8). Another source of stress may be the grandmother's desire to free herself of the constraints of being a grandmother: "If it's illness or something like that, I'd have to [help], I would [help]... But I don't think I'd do it by choice, just to suit them, because I like freedom as well" (Cotterill, 1992, p. 613). Finally, with regard to the feelings of stress that undermine the consensus of happy grandmotherhood, Robertson (1977) revealed that the role of grandmother is not significantly related to life satisfaction. In fact, the findings of Robertson's (1977) study were consistent with Blau (1973), who argued that "when in need, one good friend is more important in maintaining morale than a dozen grandchildren" (Johnson, 1983, p. 549). Evidently, there is no longer a consensus that grandmotherhood is all good. The increasing emphasis on freedom of expression, openness, and breaking myths has enabled women to develop a more balanced, complex, and diverse perspective of grandmotherhood.

The Transition to Grandmotherhood in Midlife

One of the most typical characteristics of the transition to grandparenthood is that it is initiated by someone else (i.e., the son or daughter) and is not controlled by the individual. In that sense, the transition to grandparenthood can be likened to events such as becoming an orphan or a widow, as opposed to events such as marriage or childbirth, which are self-initiated.

There are two main types of transition to grandmotherhood: off-time and on-time (Burton & Bengston, 1985). The off-time transition is not a scheduled or predictable event, as in the case of teenage pregnancy, which can lead to grandparenthood in the 30s. Becoming a grandparent "off-time" can generate numerous stressors, such as overload, obstruction of plans, conflict with the normal developmental process, and lack of a peer group (Burton et al., 1995).

In this chapter, I deal with on-time grandparenthood, which is an expected transition that usually takes place in midlife between the ages of 45 and 50, in tandem with the normative life cycle (Burton & Bengston, 1985; Matthews & Sprey, 1984). The transition to grandparenthood is one of the most comprehensive ones for the family, and it influences the roles of all family members. In the process of this life transition, family members do not give up or lose their former family roles. Rather, they add new roles to existing ones. The "child" becomes a parent, the mother or mother-in-law becomes a grandmother, and the grandparents become great grandparents. Moreover, the birth of a grandchild adds new roles to the family, such as niece and cousin.

When the transition to grandparenthood occurs at a developmentally appropriate period for both the grandparent and the adult children, then the status of grandparent is a source of identification that usually generates satisfaction (Kivett, 1998). The normative transition to grandmotherhood is not a uniform process, and is affected by social, personal, and interpersonal contexts in which it occurs. To understand the impact of the grandparenting experience, it is essential to examine events that occur in each of these contexts (Elder, 1994).

Personal Context

Regarding the personal context that may affect the transition to grandparenthood, researchers (Kivett, 1998) have mentioned the grandmother's health as a major factor. Grandparents who are in relatively good health adapt better to the transition than do those who are in poor health. Another personal factor that may affect the experience of grandparenthood is economic status. Grandparents who are experiencing financial problems buy fewer presents for their grandchildren, and do not invest as much in telephone calls and visits (Troll, 1985). Clearly, this affects the relationships between grandparents and their grandchildren.

Finally, synchronous events may work within a personal context to produce changes in the structure and function of the grandparent role (Troll, 1985). For example, grandparenthood might coincide with a midlife career change, which would have a strong impact on the grandparenting experience. Specifically, the time, effort, and resources that career changes demand detract from the investment in relations with grandchildren. Another personal context factor that can affect the transition to grandparenthood is the extent of socialization to the grandparent role. Both intense and gradual socialization can enhance role identity and performance (George, 1980). Similarly, first-time grandparents better understand the dynamics of the role if their peers are also experiencing it (for a review, see Kivett, 1998). In addition, advancements in medical technology enable grandparents to experience a process of anticipatory socialization. Today, for example, it is possible to determine the sex of the child and see pictures of the fetus during the course of the pregnancy, so that grandparents can begin developing a relationship with the grandchild even before the birth takes place.

Interpersonal Context

Relationships with other family members and with grandchildren can also affect the transition to grandparenthood. In this connection, researchers have found that the characteristics of the grandchild affect the grandparenting experience. For example, chronically ill grandchildren may intensify the involvement of grandparents in caregiving and provision of other resources (Dilworth-Anderson, 1994). Furthermore, certain social problems experienced by adult children today may affect the grandparenting role. Unexpected roles that grandparents assume as a result of social and economic crises, such as cases of alcoholism among adult children, can be a source of considerable stress (Bahr, 1994). In addition, the grandparents often intensify their involvement in the grandparenting role when their children experience economic problems, such as marginal employment or unemployment (Dressel & Barnhill, 1994).

Conversely, the experience of grandparenthood can also be affected by the way the offspring treat their grandparents. A study by Cotterill (1992) revealed that most women consider the child's grandparents to be the best source of childcare, although they would rather receive such assistance from their own mother than from their mother-in-law. Evidently, when it comes to childcare, young women share more in common with their mothers than with their mothers-in-law.

Social Context

Social context affects the transition to grandmotherhood, as well as the experience and expectations of being a grandmother. One of the main characteristics of the social context is ethnicity, which affects perspectives of grandparenthood and the symbolism attached to being a grandparent (Schlesinger & Schlesinger, 1998). For example, studies have compared the experience of grandparenting among African Americans and European Americans. Storm and Storm (1993) investigated grandparents' and grandchildren's perceptions of the grandparent role, and found that African American grandparents view the role of teacher as one of their major strengths. In that capacity, grandparents teach their children consideration of others, good manners, how to distinguish right from wrong, and religious faith. By the same token, the grandchildren also indicated that having a grandparent as a teacher is important. Thus, African American grandparents and grandchildren tend to perceive the grandparent role as more important than do their European American counterparts (Storm & Storm, 1993). Specifically, among African Americans, grandparents hold a position of authority and provide discipline and guidance. Kennedy's study of Black and White college students also revealed racial differences in expectations of grandparents' role behavior (Kennedy, 1990). Blacks were more likely than Whites to argue that grandparents help with parenting and provide financial assistance and that grandchildren should follow the guidance of grandparents. In contrast, Whites were more likely to agree that it is important to visit grandparents and share information about their activities. Whites were also more likely to differentiate between the parent and grandparent roles (e.g., grandparents should not spoil grandchildren, and grandparents should maintain contact but leave parenting to parents).

In the multicultural context of Israeli society, which integrates a wide variety of ethnic and national groups, the impact of ethnicity on grandmotherhood is particularly significant. For example, among Israeli Arabs and Jews of Asian-African origin, who are characterized by a familistic and collectivist orientation, grandparents are respected and receive more support from their children and grandchildren than do their counterparts from Western, individualist cultures. Furthermore, among immigrants who arrived in Israel from the Former Soviet Union during the last decade, the *babushka* [grandmother] receives a lot of love and respect. In fact, among recent immigrants from the Former Soviet Union, grandparents often share an apartment with their children and grandchildren as a continuation of living patterns in their country of origin, on the one hand, and economic strain in the country of immigration, on the other (Israel Central Bureau of Statistics, 2005). Therefore, grandparents are often perceived as an integral part of the nuclear family and are treated accordingly. It is the combination of personal, interpersonal, and social elements that gives the experience of midlife grandmotherhood its special, symbolic meaning.

Grandmothers in Their 50s: Acrobats with Many Hats

Today, grandmothers in their 50s are different from their own grandmothers and even from their own mothers. They are more empowered because they are healthier, more educated, younger looking, more fashionable, and more informed

(Kornhaber, 1996). In addition, they expect more of themselves, and their quality of life is usually better. Today, grandmotherhood is no longer a single commitment, and many grandmothers in their 50s are full-time workers and career women. Thus, grandmothers in their 50s fulfill more social roles than in the past—not only compared with women their age in previous generations, but also compared with the roles they fulfilled at previous stages in their own lives. Indeed, Hall's classic study on the number of roles that women perform during the life cycle revealed that in middle age women fulfill more roles than at any other stage of life (Hall, 1975).

In light of the rapid changes in the modern world, and following the general increase in longevity in the Western world, as described above, care of aging parents continues for a long period of the woman's life. In Israel, especially among the religious community and among Jews of Asian-African origin, responsibility for care of elderly members of the extended family (e.g., the father-in-law or mother-in-law) often falls squarely on the woman's shoulders (Izraeli, 1994). Thus, the traditional caregiving role that women assume in midlife is broader than at any time in the past, or at any other stage of the life cycle. In the contemporary era, it is possible that at age 50 a woman will have to care for her aging parents—a responsibility which is physically and emotionally taxing in itself—in addition to caring for children who are living at home (and sometimes are still very young), and assisting children who have left the home. Furthermore, in Israel many women at about age 50 have children serving in the army—a role that is stressful in itself. In the best of cases, being a parent to a soldier involves a considerable amount of domestic work, such as doing laundry, cooking, and ironing when the son or daughter spends weekends on leave (Izraeli, 1999). Moreover, the perpetual state of military tension in Israel is an especially significant stressor for parents of young men serving in combat units. All of this tension is compounded when the same woman is a grandmother, and is asked to care for her grandchildren so that the "younger generation" will be able to advance in their own careers. A study (Kornhaber, 1996) conducted in the United States revealed that over 3.2 million children had grandparents who were surrogate (full-time) parents. Although the situation in which grandparents replace the parents is an extreme one, grandparents often find themselves "on standby" in case they are called on to care for their grandchildren and relieve the parents of that burden. Thus, that burden often falls on the shoulders of the grandmother.

In addition to their multiple and simultaneous family roles, women who are grandmothers in their 50s also have a wide range of social roles. In many cases, at this stage of life women are at the peak of their careers after years of intensive efforts and hard work. Often, because of the changes in their lives and in their perspectives (e.g., the "empty nest" effect, changes in time perspective), women in their 50s may decide to give their careers an extra push. Midlife changes and evaluations can also provide an incentive for new activities such as going back to school, taking courses, developing a hobby they always wanted to pursue (even to the point of learning a new profession), or making a career of volunteer activities (Lieber, 1990).

Researchers (e.g., Friedman, 1987) have argued that the woman's power increases in midlife as marital power relations begin to shift. There are various explanations for the reported shift in power with age. Neugarten (1968) argued that it reflects a reversal of gender roles with age, as older men become more feminine and older women become more masculine. Expanding on this argument, Gutmann (1987) claimed that biologically determined reproductive capacities cause different aspects of the personality to be expressed or suppressed by each sex. Although both men and women have the potential to be nurturing and powerful, Gutmann (1987) referred to the "parental emergency," which forces women to develop characteristics of empathy, compassion, and nurturing. At the end of the "parental emergency" women can express aspects of themselves that they had suppressed. In a similar vein, Jung (1971) suggested that women become more masculine in middle age out of a desire to express latent personality traits. Alternatively, Rossi (1980) claimed that the increase in women's power is a result of biological changes, and other researchers have emphasized the role of psychosocial factors as reflected in changing marital, family, and social dynamics (for a review, see Friedman & Todd, 1994). In that connection, it can be argued that middle-aged grandmothers should take advantage of this shift in power because they have to be strong and develop appropriate skills for coping with simultaneous and multiple roles in contemporary society.

Thus, grandmothers in their 50s are like acrobats who juggle many roles, such as mother, wife, mother-in-law, grandmother, community volunteer, career woman, student. Often they change hats at different times of the day, depending on which role they are playing. However, there are times when they have to wear all of their hats at one time. Juggling roles without letting any of the hats drop is an art in itself. The effort and courage required to perform all of these roles successfully is truly a heroic feat.

Conclusion

This chapter provides an overview of grandparenthood in the contemporary era, with emphasis on middle-aged grandmothers in their 50s. The characteristics of grandmothers in that age group derive partly from developments in the modern era, and partly from the psychosocial processes that typify midlife. As shown here, some of the salient characteristics of grandmothers in their 50s include a variety of grandmothering styles, which differ from the image of the traditional grandmother. The diverse range of grandmothering styles derives from the relationship between the grandmothering role and the other roles that many women fulfill in midlife. In contrast to the traditional grandmothering style that prevailed in the past, which focuses on the relationship with grandchildren, the modern grandmothering style is a product of the relationship between the grandmother role (which is one dimension) and other roles such as career, leisure activities, and volunteer work.

Today, middle-aged grandmotherhood among women in their 50s can be portrayed through a gallery of images, where grandmothers have more freedom and legitimacy to choose the image or style that is appropriate for them. Because middle-aged grandmothers have many years of life ahead of them, they attempt to give those years meaning and content in various ways. Some women adhere to the traditional grandmother image and devote themselves to their grandchildren. However, of the diverse range of styles that they can adopt, they may choose alternative patterns that are more appropriate for them. In this connection, Goodfellow (2003) adopted Hakin's "preference theory" to explain grandmothers' choices of styles (Hakin, 2000). Hakin (2000), who considered the lifestyle choices of working women, proposed that women today are in a position to make a real choice between work and family when they decide to adopt a lifestyle. Preference theory focuses on women's choices in relation to work, family, and the nature of decisions about lifestyle. Consistent with preference theory, it can be argued that today middle-aged grandparents are freer than they have ever been in the past to choose the style of grandparenting that they prefer. Even women with no children (or grandchildren) who aspire to this role can choose to "adopt" neighborhood children with no grandparents (or none nearby), or, in the United States, to join an organization such as "Foster Grandparents," which matches children with older people.

In sum, one of the major conclusions of this review is that grandmothers in their 50s no longer have to conform to a homogeneous image. The diversity that characterizes numerous roles and phenomena in the contemporary era also applies to grandmotherhood. Notably, the grandmother role is integrated with other roles that women fulfill in midlife, and the possible combinations are infinite. Thus, the weight that women allocate to the grandmother role within the role set can vary, and every woman is free to create the grandmothering style that is appropriate for her.

Recommendations for Future Research

In light of the complexity of grandmotherhood today and the rapid changes that have occurred in the contemporary era, there is a need for extensive research on current developments in this area. In this context, several main research directions should be emphasized in future studies. First, there is a lack of research on grandmotherhood as a life transition among women in their 50s. The changes that have occurred in the status of middle-aged women in the contemporary era have been examined extensively from biological, psychological, and occupational perspectives. However, grandparenthood as a life transition has not been addressed sufficiently. This transition evokes intense emotions, and it involves conflicting processes, such as closure versus new beginnings, and loss versus hope and challenges. In light of the diverse range of grandmothering styles, it is important to examine the symbolic meaning of this transition to women who become grandmothers. In addition, it would be worthwhile to develop new typologies that reflect the different styles of grandmotherhood. These typologies should go beyond the traditional dimension of grandmother–grandchild relations and to examine dimensions that derive from the other roles that women fulfill in midlife.

Finally, an interesting direction for research would be the impact of the grandfather role on men in their 50s and styles of grandfatherhood at that life stage. Public and academic discourse has dealt extensively with changes in masculine roles, including the role of "new father" (Laqueur, 1992; Marsiglio, 1993). In the same vein, it can be argued that there is a "new grandfather," who expresses more emotions and is more involved with his grandchildren than grandfathers were in the past. On the one hand, there is more legitimation for men to express emotions and feelings. On the other hand, middle-aged men today often have more free time due to early retirement and a shorter work week. Thus, grandfathers can be more involved and spend more quality time with their grandchildren. Therefore, it would be worthwhile to examine the impact of "new grandfatherhood" on the role of grandmothers in their 50s. On the whole, a lot remains to be learned about grandparenthood in general and grandmotherhood in particular. In that sense, the field poses new and diverse challenges to researchers as well as to practitioners.

References

Bahr, K.S. (1994). The strengths of Apache grandmothers: Observations on commitment culture and caretaking. *Journal of Comparative Family Studies, 25*, 233–248.

Barranti, C.C.R. (1985). The grandparent/grandchild relationship: Family resources in an era of voluntary bonds. *Family Relations, 34*, 343–351.

Bastida, E. (1987). Sex-typed age norms among older Hispanics. *Gerontologist, 27*, 29–60.

Blau, Z.S. (1973). *Old Age in a Changing Society.* New York: New Viewpoints.

Boyd, R. (1967). The emerging social roles of the four-generation family. In G. Dockes (Ed.), *Our Elderly Americans: Challenge and Response* (pp. 11–21). Spartenburg, SC: Converse College Press.

Burton, L.M. (1992). Black grandparents rearing children of drug-addicted parents: Stressors, outcomes, and social service needs. *Gerontologist, 32*, 744–751.

Burton, L.M., and Bengston, V.L. (1985). Black grandmothers: Issues of timing and continuity of roles. In V.L. Bengston and J.F. Robertson (Eds.), *Grandparenthood* (pp. 61–77). Beverly Hills, CA: Sage.

Burton, L.M., Dilworth-Anderson, P., and Merriwether-deVries, C. (1995). Context and surrogate parenting among contemporary grandparents. *Marriage and Family Review, 20*, 349–366.

Cherlin, A.J., and Furstenberg, F.F. (1985). Styles and strategies of grandparenting. In V.L. Bengtson and J.F. Robertson (Eds.), *Grandparenthood* (pp. 97–116). Beverly Hills, CA: Sage.

Clavan, S. (1978). The impact of social class and social trends on the role of the grandparent. *Family Coordinator, 27*, 351–357.

Cohler, B.J., and Gruenbaum, H.V. (1981). *Mothers, Grandmothers, and Daughters: Personality and Child Care in Three Generations.* New York: Wiley.

Cotterill, P. (1992). But for freedom, you see, not to be a babyminder: Women's attitudes toward grandmother care. *Sociology, 26*, 603–618.

Creighton, L. (1991, December 16). The silent saviors. *US News & World Report*, pp. 80–89.

Denham, T.E., and Smith, C.W. (1989). The influence of grandparents on grandchildren: A review of the literature and resources. *Family Relations, 38*, 345–350.
Deutsch, H. (1945). *The Psychology of Women*. New York: Grune & Stratton.
Dilworth-Anderson, P. (1994). The importance of grandparents in extended kin caregiving to Black children with sickle cell disease. *Journal of Health and Social Policy, 5*, 185–202.
Dressel, P.L., and Barnhill, S.K. (1994). Reframing gerontological thought and practice: The case of grandmothers with daughters in prison. *Gerontologist, 34*, 685–691.
Elder, G.H. (1994). Time, human aging, and social change: Perspective on the life course. *Social Psychology Quarterly, 57*, 4–15.
Friedman, A. (1987). Getting stronger with age: Changes in women over the life cycle. *Israel Social Science Research, 5*, 76–86.
Friedman, A., and Todd, J. (1994). Kenyan women tell a story: Interpersonal power of women in three subcultures in Kenya. *Sex Roles, 31*, 503–525.
George, L.K. (1980). *Role Transitions in Later Life*. Monterey, CA: Brooks/Cole.
Giarrusso, R., Silverstein, M., and Bengston, V.L. (1996). Family complexity and the grandparent role. *Generations, 20*, 17–23.
Goodfellow, J. (2003, May). *Grandparents' Caring for Their Children's Children*. Paper presented at the Conference on Our Children: The Future, Sydney, Australia.
Gutmann, D.L. (1975). Parenthood: A key to the comparative study of life cycle. In N. Dotan and L.H. Ginzberg (Eds.), *Life Development Psychology: Normative Life Crises* (pp. 167–184). New York: Academic Press.
Gutmann, D.L. (1987). *Reclaimed Power: Toward a New Psychology of Men and Women in Later Life*. New York: Basic Books.
Hagestad, G.O. (1985). Continuity and connectedness. In V.L. Bengston and J.F. Robertson (Eds.), *Grandparenthood* (pp. 31–48). Beverly Hills, CA: Sage.
Hakin, C. (2000). *Work-lifestyle Choices in the 21st Century: Preference Theory*. London: Oxford University Press.
Hall, T. (1975). Pressures from work, self, and home in the life stages of married women. *Journal of Vocational Behavior, 6*, 127–135.
Israel Central Bureau of Statistics. (2005). *Household expenditure survey 2000–2002: Households of immigrants from the USSR (former)*. [Special Publication No. 1231]. Jerusalem: Author.
Izraeli, D.N. (1994). Money matters: Spousal income and family/work relations among physician couples in Israel. *Sociological Quarterly, 35*, 69–84.
Izraeli, D.N. (1999). Hamigdur beolam ha'avoda [Genderizing in the work place]. In D.N. Izraeli, A. Friedman, H. Dahan-Kalev, S. Fogiel-Bijaoui, H. Herzog, N. Hasan, and H. Naveh (Eds.), *Sex, Gender, Politics: Women in Israel* (pp. 167–216). Tel Aviv: Hakibbutz Hameuchad (in Hebrew).
Jannelli, L.M. (1988). Depictions of grandparents in children's literature. *Educational Gerontology, 14*, 193–202.
Johnson, C.L. (1983). A cultural analysis of the grandmother. *Research on Aging, 5*, 547–567.
Jung, C.V. (1971). The stage of life. In J. Campbell (Ed.), *The Portable Jung* (pp. 3–22). New York: Viking Press.
Kahana, B., and Kahana, E. (1971). Theoretical and research perspective on grandparenthood. *Aging and Human Development, 2*, 61–68.

Kennedy, G.E. (1990). College students' expectations of grandparent and grandchild behavior. *Gerontologist, 30*, 43–48.
Kivett, V.R. (1998). Transitions in grandparents' lives: Effects on the grandparent role. In M.E. Szinovacz (Ed.), *Handbook of Grandparenting* (pp. 131–143). Westport, CT: Greenwood Press.
Kornhaber, A. (1996). *Contemporary Grandparenting*. Thousand Oaks, CA: Sage.
Kornhaber, A., and Woodward, K. (1981). *Grandparents, Grandchildren: The Vital Connection*. Garden City, NY: Doubleday/Anchor Press.
Kulik, L. (2005). *Being a Grandmother in 2000*. Unpublished manuscript.
Lajewski, H.C. (1959). Working mothers and their arrangements for the care of their children. *Social Security Bulletin, 22*, 8–13.
Laqueur, T.W. (1992). The facts of fatherhood. In B. Throne and M. Yalom (Eds.), *Rethinking the Family: Some Feminist Questions* (pp. 155–175). Boston: Northeastern University Press.
Lieber, M. (1990). Shinui kariera be'emtza hahyim [Changing careers in mid-life]. Unpublished Master's thesis, Tel Aviv University (in Hebrew).
Marsiglio, W. (1993). Contemporary scholarship on fatherhood: Culture, identity, and conduct. *Journal of Family Issues, 14*, 484–509.
Matthews, S., and Sprey, J. (1984). The impact of divorce on grandparenting: An exploratory study. *Gerontologist, 24*, 41–47.
Minkler, M., and Roe, K.M. (1993). *Grandmothers as Caregivers*. Newbury Park, CA: Sage.
Neugarten, B. (1968). *Middle Age and Aging: A Reader in Social Psychology*. Chicago: University of Chicago Press.
Neugarten, B., and Weinstein, K. (1964). The changing American grandparent. *Journal of Marriage and the Family, 26*, 199–204.
Orbach, Z. (2001). *Savta bejeans [Grandma in jeans]*. Tel Aviv: Orbach Press (in Hebrew).
Robertson, J.F. (1976). Significance of grandparents' perceptions of young adult grandchildren. *Gerontologist, 16*, 137–140.
Robertson, J.F. (1977). Grandmotherhood: A study of role conceptions. *Journal of Marriage and the Family, 39*, 165–174.
Rossi, A. (1980). Life-span theories and women's life. *Signs, 6*, 4–32.
Schlesinger, R., and Schlesinger, B. (1998). Grandparenthood: Multiculural perspectives. *Journal of Psychology and Judaism, 22*, 247–264.
Smith, P.K. (1995). Grandparenthood. In M.H. Bornstein (Ed.), *Handbook of Parenting* (pp. 89–111). Mahwah, NJ: Erlbaum.
Storm, R., and Storm, S.K. (1993). Grandparents raising grandchildren: Goals and support groups. *Educational Gerontology, 19*, 705–715.
Sussman, M.B. (1953). The help pattern in the middle class family. *American Sociological Review, 18*, 22–28.
Sussman, M.B. (1962). Kin family network: Unheralded structural current conceptualizations of family functioning. *Marriage and Family Living, 24*, 231–240.
Timberlake, E.M. (1986). The value of grandchildren to grandmothers. *Journal of Gerontological Social Work, 2*, 63–67.
Troll, L.E. (1983). Grandparents: The party watchdogs. In T. Brubaker (Ed.), *Family Relationships in Later Life* (pp. 67–74). Beverly Hills, CA: Sage.
Troll, L.E. (1985). The contingencies of grandparenting. In V.L. Bengston and J.F. Robertson (Eds.), *Grandparenthood* (pp. 135–149). Beverly Hills, CA: Sage.

Uhlenberg, P., and Kirby, J.B. (1998). Grandparenthood over time: Historical and demographic trends. In M.E. Szinovacz (Ed.), *Handbook on Grandparenthood* (pp. 23–39). Westport, CT: Greenwood Press.

Werner, E.E. (1991). Grandparent–grandchild relationships among US ethnic groups. In P.K. Smith (Ed.), *The Psychology of Grandparenthood: An International Perspective* (pp. 68–82). London: Routledge & Kegan Paul.

Young, M. (1959). The role of the extend family in disaster. *Human Relations, 7*, 189–204.

8
Women Over 50: Caregiving Issues

Rosalie J. Ackerman and Martha E. Banks

Tina[1], on caregiving for her father:

Does all caregiving begin with a telephone call? Mine did.
  Tina (mid 30s): "Happy Birthday to You, Happy Birthday to You, Happy Birthday, Dear..."
  Father (early 60s): "I've got cancer."
  The first call led to caregiving by my mother, then in her mid 60s. My father's cancer was diagnosed late, despite his semiannual checkups. As a result, my mother found herself having to provide caregiving at home. The initial prognosis of 6 weeks was wrong; my father lived for another 16 months. During his illness, my mother cared for him at home as long as she could. My siblings and I visited, but we were serving supportive roles with my mother clearly being the primary caregiver. After a year, she enlisted the assistance of her sister, also in her mid 60s, who flew to the United States from Barbados, West Indies to help for as long as necessary. The two of them soon found that they could not manage and asked me to come home. After 2 days, it was clear that the three of us could not provide all of the care my father needed. Nursing assistance was not available, and the oncologist arranged for my father's care in a nursing home. My mother stayed by his side for about 18 hours a day until he died. My mother had severely limited her social network activities while attending to her husband's medical needs.
  Caregiving can involve loss of familiar ways of relating. My family thrived on our intellect. We debated and discussed, priding ourselves on our educational accomplishments (my parents pursued and received their Master's degrees while I was in college and graduate school). Caregiving involved losing the stimulating conversation and their proud support of my accomplishments and those of my siblings; I was not prepared for that loss while my parents were alive. I was also unprepared for my father's anger and extreme disappointment with the unplanned nursing home placement.
  Was my mother prepared for caregiving for an adult? For many years, my mother was a geriatric social worker who assisted families in securing assistance for caregiving. She was briefly a member of the "sandwich generation" during her mid 40s when my paternal grandmother, who lived with us, was diagnosed with cancer. My grandmother's diagnosis was so late that she lived only a few weeks beyond diagnosis. My mother cared for her

---
[1] Pseudonym

at home for about 2 or 3 weeks before my grandmother's final hospitalization. During the previous 2 years, my mother's father and then her mother had died. My mother was unable to spend time with her father before he died, and she saw her mother only briefly before life support was removed. Her sister, single, in her mid 40s, and living with my grandparents, had provided care for my grandparents at home in Saint Vincent, West Indies where she had had the assistance of servants and nurses. When my mother called my aunt, then also in her mid 60s, to help with my father, my aunt was a relative expert at physical caregiving for ill adults.

Was I prepared for caregiving for an adult? Although I was in clinical practice in a geriatric rehabilitation facility, I was not at all prepared to care for my father. The personal assistance I observed 5 days a week was provided by a trained multidisciplinary staff. In my parents' home, three untrained women were not appropriately prepared to take care of my father.

In my family, on both sides, despite the differences in national backgrounds, eldest daughters were historically expected to be the family caregivers. As a child, I had observed some of my paternal grandmother's elderly cousins providing care for other elderly relatives. I assumed they learned from each other as part of a large extended family living in close proximity to each other. I grew up in a nuclear family that included my paternal grandmother; there were no extended family members in the same state. At the time of my father's illness, I was a single eldest daughter with a career. I was pressured by some distant relatives to give up the career and devote my full efforts to my father's care.

My best contribution to my father's care was my ability to talk with the healthcare professionals and to facilitate their direct communication with my father. In addition, I was able to assist in his pain management. He tried to follow a schedule for his pain medication in order to avoid addiction. As a result, he had cycles of terrible pain. I explained that he needed to take the medicine more often in order to control the pain; again, I interceded with the oncologist for better explanation that "prn (as needed)" superceded the schedule listed on the prescription.

Sometimes, caregiving ends with a telephone call. Mine did.

    Tina's Sister (mid 20s): Daddy just passed away.

The level of my mother's grief when my father died was reflective, in part, of a disbelief that such a thing could happen. She was as unprepared for the end of caregiving as she was for the personal assistance during caregiving.

Becky[2], on caregiving for her friend:

During my early 50s, I served as a caregiver for a friend following emergency surgery. Although I had anticipated that I would be providing mere living space for 1 or 2 weeks, I was a caregiver for about 6 months. My home was on one level, and my friend was unable to manage the stairs in her house. When I made the offer of my home, I did not realize how ill my friend would be. I had assumed that she would be able to take care of herself when she was released from the hospital. Instead, she needed assistance with meals and transportation to medical appointments. I also had to assist in some medical decisions. Because I had not planned to provide that level of care, and found that I had to juggle my job and social life with her care, it created a strain on our friendship. I was angry, but had no suitable target for my anger.

---

[2] Pseudonym

Tina, on caregiving for her mother:

Caregiving onset phone call:
Mother (late 60s): "I went for my daily drive and got lost coming home."

Years later, when I got the call from my mother, I, then in my early 40s, was better prepared than when my father was ill. My mother helped in that preparation by writing a living will with very specific directives about her desires for care and living situations. If I followed my mother's directives, I would not be responsible for physical personal assistance myself, but instead for the monitoring of professionals in an alternative setting.

Caregiving for my mother was a shared responsibility, with my siblings taking the first turns as primary caregivers. Throughout the process, my siblings and I supported each others' caregiving efforts. My caregiving contributions for my mother varied across the years and included some personal assistance; emotional support; arrangement for medical assessments, living situations, and healthcare; monitoring progress; and training and retraining treatment staff. Despite following her wishes, I struggled with the amount of monitoring that I should do to ensure that my mother received appropriate physical care.

When my mother's death was clearly imminent for 2 days, I found myself struggling with shock that she was really going to die, disappointment in myself as a healthcare professional that I could not stop her from dying, and conflict about what others might think of my supporting my mother's request for no extraordinary measures, as her death occurred a few weeks after the media, Congress, and the Supreme Court involved themselves in Terry Schiavo's death. However, it was only during that period of imminent death that I was able to say goodbye and openly grieve in her presence.

I left my mother's nursing home briefly to grab a bite of supper. As I got in the car, Mozart's Requiem *was on the radio. I commented, "How did they know?" Later as I started to prepare supper and call my sister to give her an update, my other phone rang.*

Nurse: I'm sorry to inform you that your mother just died.

Family caregivers wrestle not only with tasks, but with fundamental questions of life, their own mortality, as well as with relationships with people important to them, who may be suffering and dying (Ziemba & Lynch-Sauer, 2005, p. 111).

What Is Caregiving?

Caregiving involves direct personal assistance [assistance with activities of daily living (ADLs[3]) and instrumental activities of daily living (IADLs[4])], as well as primary responsibility for the health and welfare of people receiving informal care

---

[3] "Activities of daily living are activities related to personal care and include bathing or showering, dressing, getting in or out of bed or a chair, using the toilet, and eating" (US Department of Health and Human Services, Centers for Disease Control and Prevention, National Center for Health Statistics, 2004a).

[4] "Instrumental activities of daily living are activities related to independent living and include preparing meals, managing money, shopping for groceries or personal items, performing light or heavy housework, and using a telephone" (US Department of Health and Human Services, Centers for Disease Control and Prevention, National Center for Health Statistics, 2004b).

in the community or formal care in institutions. Many women over the age of 50 provide caregiving. This issue is of concern to women because they disproportionately care for others (Adams et al., 2002; Banks & Ackerman, 2006; Browder, 2002; Farran, 1997; Fuller-Thomson, 2005; Hunt, 2003; Kiecolt-Glaser & Newton, 2001; Minkler, 2005; Minkler & Fuller-Thomson, 2005; Sleath et al., 2005; US Census Bureau, 2004a; 2004b). In addition, there is some evidence that the caregiving process negatively affects women's health more severely and for longer periods than it does for men (Vahtera et al., 2006). Some of the issues faced by women caring for parents, adult children, grandchildren, significant others, and friends include ways in which they find themselves in the role of caregiver, preparation for caregiving, variety of family roles, support and self-care, harm in the caregiving relationship, and loss during and at the end of caregiving.

The term "caregiving" has been perceived by some to indicate passive provision and receipt of care (Mona, 2003), however, caregiving involves an active relationship. For this chapter, the term "personal care assistance" is limited to situations in which the person providing the assistance does not have primary responsibility for that care. By connotation, "caregiving" excludes parenting of infants and young children. "Parenting" generally tends to be celebrated, whereas "caregiving" is often regarded as negative and burdensome. It is important, however, to consider that both "caregiving" and "parenting" involve provision of personal assistance *and* responsibility for the welfare of another person.

There has been considerable research on caregiving. Much of the research has focused on the negative impact of caregiving on caregivers. In this chapter, we will provide an overview of the positive aspects of caregiving while acknowledging the realistic difficulties engendered in the caregiving process. The research provides models of caregiving and recommendations for efficient and mutually beneficial caregiving relationships.

The Beginning of Caregiving

The examples of Tina's and Becky's caregiving illustrate clear onsets to caregiving. However, caregiving does not always have a clear beginning. In some households or communities, a member's health might gradually decline and a woman finds herself providing more and more personal assistance without considering her contributions to be caregiving. There is no clear demarcation between provision of personal assistance and caregiving, but caregiving implies a broader sense of overall responsibility than personal assistance. For example, Harland and Cuskelly (2000) described the caregiving provided by mothers of children who grew into adulthood with congenital disabilities. Siblings of those children were perceived as having limited opportunities to provide personal assistance, but the mothers were considered primary caregivers. Those siblings found themselves to be unprepared for caregiving when their mothers were no longer able to serve as caregivers.

Preparation for Caregiving

In the examples, Tina and her mother were unprepared for caregiving for Tina's father, just as Becky was not ready to be a caregiver for her friend. The experience of attempting to care for her father combined with her mother's careful planning provided a foundation for Tina later to be a caregiver for her mother.

Much of the psychological literature on caregiving examines the perceptions of caregivers on various personal assistance tasks that are part of caregiving. Attention is paid to issues of burden, resentment, and, to a lesser extent, benefits and reciprocity. A search of the caregiving literature for "preparation" primarily yielded articles and chapters on "meal preparation" as a physical care task. There is far less literature on preparation for the psychological part of caregiving. Farran (1997) also raised the question of whether caregiving involves free choice.

England and Tripp-Reimer (2003, as cited in Riley & Bowen, 2005) suggested that "a significant number of the participants in their study revealed that their behaviors and emotions represented unfavorable levels of preparedness for long-term caregiving" (p. 55). Harland and Cuskelly (2000) noted that, in many instances, transitions from one caregiver to another within families are impeded by gender role expectations. Mothers who have raised children with disabilities sometimes have difficulty relinquishing that responsibility or allowing other family members to prepare to take over the caregiving as the child moves into adulthood and the mother faces her own aging and health difficulties. Other women struggle with a lack of helpful family members and limited access to support services for the transfer of responsibility for dependent adults in need of care (Tryssenaar & Tremblay, 2002).

Ziemba and Lynch-Sauer (2005) described several psychological concerns in caregiving for parents. These include ongoing grief, dealing with multiple losses, role reversals, family role distortions, loss of parental support, and confronting one's own mortality or the end of a bloodline. Loos and Bowd (1997) described losses of social and recreational interaction, control over life events, well-being, and occupation. Ziemba and Lynch-Sauer (2005) found that caregivers felt particularly unprepared for the psychological responses to the caregiving situation, even after previous caregiving, and especially when dealing with additional grief. One issue that they did not discuss is the lack of linearity in the demands of caregiving. Although it is possible to read about the physical and cognitive declines of, for example, people with Alzheimer's dementia, it is seldom acknowledged that the decline is not steady. People have "good" days when symptoms appear to be diminished and behavior is manageable, and other days when symptoms are dramatically worse. Sometimes, the change from good to bad occurs in a matter of hours or minutes. It is very difficult to adjust to those changes; in some cases, caregivers think that the symptoms are exhibited intentionally by a person who is more in control of her or his behavior than is actually the case (Williamson et al., 2005).

Tina, for example, experienced loss of intellectual conversation with her parents as she became caregiver for the people who had provided her with care as she grew up. She missed the parental pride as she progressed in her career and faced concerns about potential life-threatening genetic vulnerabilities. Becky lost the peer-to-peer relationship while providing caregiving for her friend.

Browder (2002) noted that caregiving also involves difficult decision making (e.g., handling of finances, setting priorities, placement options, seeking assistance), some of which involve a sense of accomplishment and others of which leave caregivers struggling with options even after decisions have been made. Pain management is another extremely important issue in caregiving for people with cancer, traumatic brain injury sequelae, surgeries, and deteriorating diseases (Kiecolt-Glaser & Newton, 2001; Riley-Doucet, 2005); Tina had to intervene with her father's pain management regimen.

One area of preparation is the role of spirituality as a foundation for defining and understanding the caregiving relationship (Davis et al., 1998). Religion and spirituality also serve to decrease distress during the grief that precedes, follows, or is coincident with caregiving (Winston, 2003).

Psychologists can assist in the preparation for caregiving. Ziemba and Lynch-Sauer (2005) recommended providing potential or new caregivers with information about the time involved, resources for resolving ADL and IADL care concerns, guidance in anticipatory grief, development of "what–if" plans for predictable events, and crisis intervention for unanticipated physical and emotional reactions. As much as possible, it is useful to ensure that caregivers have adequate support networks and opportunities for relief from caregiving tasks (Banks, 2003; Banks et al., 2005; Eisdorfer et al., 2003).

Caregiving as One of Multiple Roles

In exploring caregiving by women over 50 years of age, it is useful to consider the family status of those women. Much of the literature on women as caregivers has focused on the "sandwich generation," that is, women who are taking care of elderly family members while still raising their own children in the home. This literature tends to overlook women providing care for significant others, women whose offspring are dependent adults, women with no offspring, and career women with independent adult children who, like Becky, find themselves caring for friends.

Since the end of World War II, the United States has promoted the nuclear family as a "normative" ideal. The expectation for such families is that there are two married heterosexual adults living monogamously with their minor children but without other people in the home. This "ideal" has become a stereotypic caricature of families, and most portrayals of such families are European American. The 2004 census revealed that most households differ from that nuclear family, which represents only 22% of US households (US Census Bureau, 2004a, 2004b).

African American families have, for most of the twentieth and into the twenty-first century, included nuclear, extended (includes other blood relatives, e.g., grandparents, aunts, uncles, cousins), and augmented (includes close friends, neighbors, members of social networks, e.g., religious organizations, local political groups, community-based organizations) families (Boyd-Franklin & Franklin, 2000; Hayles et al., 2004; Tatum, 1999). Jones and Shorter-Gooden (2003) described the critical role of "otherkin" in the raising of children; similar involvement of augmented family in the care of older people is less well researched, but is considered to be a supportive factor:

> the role of extended family and fictive kin is considered particularly salient, that is, the composition of the caregiving network and the likelihood that older African Americans may draw upon support beyond the nuclear family as an alternative to the use of formal services. (Cagney & Agree, 2005, p. S317)

Lesbians often have "families of choice" including partners and friends (Fredriksen, 1999). The experience and support available through such family constellations increases the opportunities for potential caregivers to be aware of and to prepare for a variety of caregiving circumstances.

Missing from these and similar studies is a tradition observed by some families in which the eldest daughters are informally designated as the family caregivers; such was the case in Tina's family of origin. In such families, the eldest daughter is single throughout her lifetime or marries when she is beyond childbearing age. Although she might have a career, she is expected to be the most available family member in the event of any family situation that would involve the need for caregiving; her career is perceived as relatively unimportant by some family members. Nabors and Pettee (2003) described the dilemma of women designated as family caregivers who found themselves only marginally supported by their families in their own times of need due to disabling physical conditions. Such women were perceived as ill only immediately following strokes or accidents, but their families were focused on how quickly the women could resume caregiving responsibilities for other family members.

Much of the literature on women caregivers over the age of 50 assumes that the women providing caregiving are heterosexual and married. Fredriksen (1999) found that, compared to gay men, lesbians were more likely to provide care for children and older adults. In addition to the many issues faced by all caregivers, "lesbian and gay caregivers may encounter limited access to partners with serious illnesses or disabilities, friends, or other family members" (Fredriksen, 1999, p. 151). Because caregiving involves formal or informal responsibility for another person, lesbians are at risk for being prevented from serving as caregivers (Riggle et al., 2005).

Some women over the age of 50 provide caregiving for adult children or siblings with disabilities (Harland & Cuskelly, 2000). Williams and Robinson (2001) described a household in which a woman provided care for her adult son and daughter who both had severe learning disabilities; she relied on both of them for assistance, for example, with getting out of the bathtub. Melberg (2005) noted similar mutual support among rural Norwegian families.

Some caregivers are conflicted between their roles as informal caregivers within their families and their professional duties as healthcare providers (Ward-Griffin, 2004). Tina, as a geropsychologist, experienced such conflict. Part of the conflict involves the unrealistic medical model that doggedly focuses on cure rather than acknowledging the reality that some disease processes are not curable and that inevitable death should not be construed as failure. An additional conflict occurs as new medications and treatments become available, leaving caregivers with decisions about the introduction of experimental treatments that might alleviate some symptoms without being actual "cures."

Grandparenting

Recent attention has been given to the increasing number of grandparents, usually grandmothers, who are raising their grandchildren. Consistent with the myth of the nuclear family is the myth of grandparents as couples sharing a pleasant retirement without the caregiving responsibilities that dominated their younger years. The reality is that nearly 6 million grandparents live in households with their grandchildren, and approximately 2.5 million grandparents are raising their grandchildren due to the unavailability of the children's parents (Minkler & Fuller-Thomson, 2005). More than one-half (62.8%) of those childrearing grandparents are women. Many of these grandparents complain of psychological burden, role overload, and lack of support. They are dealing with their own health issues, including visual and hearing problems, as well as functional limitations in their own activities of daily living. Grandmothers, who have physical problems and/or are living in poverty, have more difficulty providing caregiving for their grandchildren and experience more depression than do those in better health and with more resources (Li, 2005). For more information about grandparenting, readers are referred to the chapter by Liat Kulik (this volume).

Nature of the Caregiving Relationship

In Eurocentric societies, models of caregiving include positive and deficit or negative attributes. Some models illustrate more effective and relevant issues as well as mutuality in addressing the caregiving process (Eisdorfer et al., 2003; Farran, 1997; Kiecolt-Glaser & Newton, 2001; Lyons et al., 2002).

Farran (1997) suggested that positive aspects of caregiving are poorly defined—perhaps the terms "stress" and "positive aspects" are opposites that cannot be reconciled. Stress implies that something is wrong. An existential paradigm, on the other hand, espouses values, freedom of choice, responsibility, and consequences of actions. Values may be expressed as caregivers creatively deal with their situations.

A stress/coping paradigm most commonly asks "What does it mean to provide care to an impaired family member in terms of caregiving tasks (stress appraisal), what resources are available to caregivers, and what effect does this experience have on caregivers (outcomes)?" In an existential paradigm, one asks "How can I discover or create meaning?" (Farran, 1997, p. 254)

According to Farran (1997), several investigators have suggested that there are recurring themes that describe the caregiving process. Adaptation defines the entire process that occurs in response to the stress of caring for a person with dementia. In addition, resource variables such as coping skills, personal control, self-efficacy, knowledge, and hardiness; primary and secondary appraisal; and emotional and physical health outcomes are important. Tina found caregiving to be a means to repay her parents for raising her. Becky, in retrospect, felt a closer bond with her friend as she and her friend shared an experience that most friends do not have. They had mutual greater appreciation for each other's strengths and vulnerabilities.

In an overview of the caregiving literature, Hunt (2003) found that the predominant foci were on negative (caregiver burden, caregiver strain, or caregiver stress), positive (caregiver esteem, uplifts of caregiving, satisfaction, finding or making meaning through caregiving, or gain in the caregiving experience), and neutral (caregiver appraisal).

Farran's existential approach to understanding caregiving provides a positive framework, but much of the research concerns buffers or modifiers that make it possible for people to manage caregiving, although the focus is on the burdensome aspects of caregiving. For example, Lyons et al. (2002) noted that "[t]here is broad consensus in the caregiving literature that caring for an elderly relative places the caregiver at risk for compromised physical and mental health" (p. P195), and Gilley et al. (2005) indicated that "[t]he emotional cost of providing care to a family member with a dementia syndrome can be substantial" (p. 173). Sherwood et al. (2005) focused on the depression that can arise with the burden of caregiving.

Lyons et al. (2002) examined caregiving dyads with positive and negative attributions of the interactive context within individual relationships and in a group sample. Important comparisons were the perceptions of depression, subjective social burden, medical negative health conditions across the time span, restricted social-activity burden in both roles of caregiving, and dyadic psychological wellbeing. The dyadic relationship predicted negative outcomes of caregiver strain. Within the dyad, both caregivers and care recipients generally provided equivalent evaluations of the daily living activities and needs of care recipients. Dyads in which caregivers who reported more caregiving difficulties than care recipients did had poorer relationship quality. Coping training or other therapeutic interventions might be used to reduce the situational stress of the caregivers.

Kiecolt-Glaser and Newton (2001) developed a pathway model for aspects of caregiving in marital relationships that impacts upon physical and psychological health. They noted "that negative aspects of social relationships are often independent of positive aspects... and are important independent predictors of psychological and physical functioning" (p. 474). Li and Seltzer (2005) found a similar independence between positive (daughters' feelings of closeness to parents) and negative (daughters' sense of strain in interactions with parents) aspects of parent–daughter relationships as they impacted on daughters' self-esteem. The results of both studies suggest that reduction of the strain in relationships between caregivers and care recipients is critical to the success of the caregiving relationship.

During the process of caregiving, changes in the care recipient's health can lead to the need for changes in the living situation. For people with progressive disorders, "family caregivers are likely to be increasingly aware that institutionalization may eventually become necessary. This awareness is likely to engender some cognitive dissonance, particularly when the caregiver has negative attitudes related to institutionalization" (Gilley et al., 2005, p. 185). Tina's mother, who had been a geriatric social worker dealing with nursing home placement, assisted in her caregiving by developing a living will that stated her preference to be institutionalized as soon as she was unable to live independently. However, Tina's mother had not wanted to place her own husband in a nursing home, even when it was clear that adequate care could no longer be provided in her home.

One of the burdens of caregiving is that a family member who provides direct personal assistance has a limited opportunity to be gainfully employed. This results in increased financial pressures during a period when the care recipient, and therefore the family, is likely to be faced with high healthcare costs (Hirst, 2005). The United States has been slow to consider or implement universal health care. In one country with universal health care, Väänänen et al. (2005) found that Finnish women who perceived themselves as providing support for intimate others had low rates of work absence and better health than those who did not hold such self-perceptions. The state of Arkansas instituted a program that provided cash allowances for the purchase of personal assistance for Medicaid recipients (Simon-Rusinowitz et al., 2005). The allowances made it possible for families to hire nonspousal family members to provide assistance with ADLs and IADLs. This allowed caregivers to work fewer hours or to leave their jobs in order to provide more care than would otherwise have been possible. Simon-Rusinowitz et al. (2005) found that families often hired relatives as caregivers in the belief that they would provide better quality assistance than strangers would. There were high levels of satisfaction among caregivers and care recipients. It is important to note that family members would have served as caregivers without the financial incentive and did not feel coerced into service; this might be a reflection of the fact that 40% of the family members in the sample were African Americans, whose culture includes caring for relatives as a highly valued activity. Feld et al. (2005) found that African American spousal caregiving dyads were 63% more likely than European American spousal caregiving dyads to include other people in their caregiving networks.

Harm in the Caregiving Relationship

One of the problems in caregiving involves difficult interpersonal relations between caregivers and care recipients. In some cases involving dementia, for example, care recipients can become aggressive and injure their caregivers (Banks & Ackerman, 1992, 2002; Banks et al., 1995; Beach et al., 2005; Bruce et al., 2005; Garand et al., 2005; Sleath et al., 2005). Fultz et al. (2005) observed such aggression in men with urinary incontinence when their caregiving wives also had incontinence. Other symptoms that can lead to aggression toward caregivers include hallucinations, delusions, and confusion. Some caregivers have been the victims of intimate partner or other family violence through much of their adulthood; the violence does not always end when the perpetrator becomes a care recipient (Bergeron, 2005; Kwong et al., 2003).

In a study of increased risk of physical illness, disability problems, or mental health deterioration, Kiecolt-Glaser and Newton (2001) found that high stress with marital conflict exhibited in marriages can lessen the effectiveness of vaccines, slow wound healing, increase the risk of infectious diseases, and increase blood pressure. The stress-induced decrease in the health of caregivers impairs the ability to provide and/or oversee welfare and healthcare efficiently and beneficially.

Caregivers who perceive caregiving as a burden or who are the victims of care recipient aggression often experience depression and anxiety (Adams et al., 2002; Banks et al., 1995; Bruce et al., 2005; Rysberg, 2005). Anger toward an aggressive care recipient appears to be moderated by the caregiver's perception of the aggression as a consequence of the disease process or intentional behavior, possibly as exhibited by the recipient prior to the need for care (Williamson et al., 2005). It is important to assess behaviors of a care recipient that might negatively impact on a caregiver (e.g., irritability, confusion, inappropriate laughter, catastrophic reaction, low frustration tolerance); some recent psychological tests have incorporated evaluation for such behaviors (e.g., Ackerman-Banks Neuropsychological Rehabilitation Battery; Ackerman & Banks, 2006). Clinicians should consider neuropsychological evaluations when there is aggression in the caregiving dyad, as head injuries are possible precipitants or consequences of dyadic aggression (Ackerman & Banks, 2003, 2006; Banks, 2003; Banks & Ackerman 1992, 2002; Banks et al., 1995).

The End of Caregiving: Death and Bereavement

Also missing from the literature is the psychological impact of the end of caregiving due to death or other loss of the caregiving relationship. As Li (2005) noted, "Caregiving and bereavement are often interrelated, as most deaths of older persons in America occur after a period of chronic illness, disability, and family caregiving... The literature, however, tends to treat these events separately" (p. P190). The reality is that caregiving often coincides with a prolonged grieving period.

Caregiving of people in declining health can lead to caregivers' questioning their worldviews and struggling with the meaning of the caregiving experience as it relates to impending loss. Davis et al. (1998) found that, although "religious belief systems might make loss more comprehensible" (p. 571), those belief systems did not predict the level of distress in relation to making sense of loss or benefiting from the experience of losing a family member.

The imminence of death in the twenty-first century often evokes a decision by caregivers about the application, withholding, or withdrawal of life-sustaining treatment. Such decisions are never easy, but can be assisted, as in Tina's situation with her mother, by preplanning when the care recipient is able to participate in the decision making. Hansen et al. (2004) described the process for caregivers as involving strain or relative ease in making decisions. They noted that the sense of strain or "ease" can change prior to, during, and after the actual decision making, which can occur over an extended period of time or quickly during a sudden change in physical status. Such decision making can be further complicated by media coverage of extreme situations regarding life extension ("Terry Schiavo," 2005).

Bonanno et al. (2005) described the importance of resilience in the management of grief during and after caregiving. In some societies, the taboo about the discussion of death and an unrealistic focus on a (miracle) cure make it particularly difficult for caregivers to grieve and to share their grief with the care recipient. Tina and her mother both experienced such difficulty with openly addressing loss and handling grieving during the caregiving process.

Resources for Caregivers

There are support services available to caregiving women over the age of 50. Many women do not use those services because they do not perceive them as necessary, do not know of their availability, or cannot access them (Brodaty et al., 2005). Eisdorfer et al. (2003) examined two techniques to reduce caregiver depression: family therapy and an integrated computer–telephone communication system to enhance contact with relatives and include family members in psychotherapy.

A standard self-help book, which has been updated several times, is *The 36-Hour Day* (Mace & Rabins, 2001). For women with internet access, one resource is *Health Compass* (2005), a joint project of the American Federation for Aging Research and the Merck Institute on Aging and Health. Many states or counties have Offices on Aging or similar oversight agencies that can assist in the coordination of services. There are support groups available, often organized by disorders, such as Alzheimer's dementia. We recommend that caregivers (adapted from American Psychological Association, 2004):

- accept help and support from those who care about you and will listen to you;
- change how you interpret the circumstances that led to the need for caregiving;
- try to see beyond an immediate crisis to how future circumstances may be a little better;
- accept that change is a part of living;
- set goals for yourself and do something regularly—even if it seems like a small accomplishment—that enables you to move toward your own goals;
- establish new routines as soon as you can, even if you know they have to change in the future;
- develop an optimistic outlook that enables you to expect that good things will happen in your life. Try to keep a positive self-image;

- get regular exercise and try to find something to do that will relax you. Taking care of yourself helps to keep your mind and body primed to deal with situations that require strength;
- use meditation or other spiritual practices to build connections and restore hope.

References

Ackerman, R.J., and Banks, M.E. (2003). Assessment, treatment, and rehabilitation for interpersonal violence victims: Women sustaining head injuries. In M.E. Banks and E. Kaschak (Eds.), *Women with Visible and Invisible Disabilities: Multiple Intersections, Multiple Issues, Multiple Therapies* (pp. 343–363). New York: Haworth Press.

Ackerman, R.J., and Banks, M.E. (2006). *Manual for Administration and Interpretation for the Ackerman-Banks Neuropsychological Rehabilitation Battery© (A-BNRB, 2006 ed.).* Akron, OH: ABackans Diversified Computer Processing.

Adams, B., Aranda, M.P., Kemp, B., and Takagi, K. (2002). Ethnic and gender differences in distress among Anglo American, African American, Japanese American, and Mexican American spousal caregivers of persons with dementia. *Journal of Clinical Geropsychology, 8,* 279–301.

American Psychological Association. (2004). *The Road to Resilience.* Retrieved October 17, 2005 from http://www.apahelpcenter.org/featuredtopics/feature.php?id=6

Banks, M.E. (2003). Disability in the family: A life-span perspective. *Cultural Diversity and Ethnic Minority Psychology, 9,* 367–384.

Banks, M.E., and Ackerman, R.J. (1992). Family psychotherapy for brain-injured patients. In J.C. Chrisler and D. Howard (Eds.), *New Directions in Feminist Psychology: Practice, Theory, and Research* (pp. 66–84). New York: Springer.

Banks, M.E., and Ackerman, R.J. (2002). Head and brain injuries experienced by African American women victims of intimate partner violence. *Women & Therapy, 25*(3/4), 133–143.

Banks, M.E., and Ackerman, R.J. (2006). Health disparities: Focus on disability. In K. Hagglund and A. Heinemann (Eds.), *Advances in Disability and Rehabilitation Research* (pp. 45–70). New York: Springer.

Banks, M.E., Ackerman, R.J., and Corbett, C.A. (1995). Feminist neuropsychology: Issues for physically challenged women. In J. Chrisler and A. Hemstreet (Eds.), *Variations on a Theme: Diversity and the Psychology of Women* (pp. 29–49). Albany, NY: State University of New York Press.

Banks, M.E., Ackerman, R.J., Yee, B., and West, C. (2005). Stress and trauma in the lives of women of color. In K. Kendall-Tackett (Ed.), *The Handbook of Women, Stress, and Trauma* (pp. 207–228). New York: Brunner-Routledge.

Beach, S.R., Schultz, R., Williamson, G.M., Millar, L., Weiner, M.F., and Lance, C.E. (2005.) Risk factors for potentially harmful informal caregiver behavior. *Journal of the American Geriatrics Society, 53,* 255–261.

Bergeron, L.R. (2005). Abuse of elderly women in family relationships: Another form of violence against women In K. Kendall-Tackett (Ed.), *The Handbook of Women, Stress, and Trauma* (pp. 141–157). New York: Brunner-Routledge.

Bonanno, G.A., Moskowitz, J.T., Papa, A., and Folkman, S. (2005). Resilience to loss in bereaved spouses, bereaved parents, and bereaved gay men. *Journal of Personality and Social Psychology, 88,* 827–843.

Boyd-Franklin, N., and Franklin, A.J. (2000). *Boys into Men: Raising our African American Teenage Sons.* New York: Plume.

Brodaty, H., Thomson, C., Thompson, C., and Fine, M. (2005). Why caregivers of people with dementia and memory loss don't use services. *International Journal of Geriatric Psychiatry, 20,* 537–546.

Browder, S. (2002). "My mind's made up": Assumptions and decision-making in accounts of caregiving women. *Journal of Women & Aging, 14*(3/4), 77–97.

Bruce, D.G., Paley, G.A., Nichols, P., Roberts, D., Underwood, P.J., and Schaper, F. (2005). Physical disability contributes to caregiver stress in dementia caregivers. *Journals of Gerontology: Series A: Biological Sciences and Medical Sciences, 60A,* 345–349.

Cagney, K.A., and Agree, E.M (2005). Racial differences in formal long-term care: Does the timing of parenthood play a role? *Journals of Gerontology: Series B: Psychological Sciences and Social Sciences, 60B,* S137–S145.

Davis, C.G., Nolen-Hoeksema, S., and Larson, J. (1998). Making sense of loss and benefiting from the experience: Two construals of meaning. *Journal of Personality and Social Psychology, 75,* 561–574.

Eisdorfer, C., Czaja, S.J., Loewenstein, D.A., Rubert, M.P., Arguelles, S., Mitrani, V.B., and Szapocznik, J. (2003). The effect of a family therapy and technology-based intervention on caregiver depression. *Gerontologist, 43,* 521–531.

Farran, C.J. (1997). Theoretical perspectives concerning positive aspects of caring for elderly persons with dementia: Stress/adaptation and existentialism. *Gerontologist, 37,* 250–258.

Feld, S., Dunkle, R.E., and Schroepfer, T. (2005). When do couples expand their ADL caregiver network beyond the marital dyad? *Marriage and Family Review, 37,* 27–44.

Fredriksen, K.I. (1999). Family caregiving responsibilities among lesbians and gay men. *Social Work, 44,* 142–155.

Fuller-Thomson, E. (2005). Canadian First Nations grandparents raising grandchildren: A portrait in resilience. *International Journal of Aging and Human Development, 60,* 331–342.

Fultz, N.H., Jenkins, K.R., Ostbye, T., Taylor, D.H., Kabeto, M.U., and Langa, K.M. (2005). The impact of own and spouse's urinary incontinence on depressive symptoms. *Social Science and Medicine, 60,* 2537–2548.

Garand, L., Dew, M.A., Eazor, L.R., DeKosky, S.T., and Reynolds, C.F. (2005). Caregiving burden and psychiatric morbidity in spouses of with mild cognitive impairment. *International Journal of Geriatric Psychiatry, 20,* 512–522.

Gilley, D.W., McCann, J.J., Bienias, J.L., and Evans, D.A. (2005). Caregiver psychological adjustment and institutionalization of persons with Alzheimer's disease. *Journal of Aging and Health, 17,* 172–189.

Hansen, L, Archbold, P.G., and Stewart, B.J. (2004). Role strain and ease in decision-making to withdraw or withhold life support for elderly relatives. *Journal of Nursing Scholarship, 36,* 233–238.

Harland, P., and Cuskelly, M. (2000). The responsibilities of adult siblings of adults with dual sensory impairments. *International Journal of Disability, Development, and Education, 47,* 293–307.

Hayles, V.R., Jr., Bell, S.R., Evans, W., Floyd, L.J., Monteiro, N., Daniels, I.N., and Harrell, C.J.P. (2004). African American strengths: A selective contemporary review. In R.L. Jones (Ed.), *Black Psychology* (4th ed., pp. 405–425). Hampton, VA: Cobb & Henry.

Health Compass: Navigating Research Information on Aging and Health. (2005). Retrieved October 17, 2005 from http://www.healthcompass.org/

Hirst, M. (2005). Carer distress: A prospective, population-based study. *Social Science and Medicine, 61*, 697–708.

Hunt, C.K. (2003). Concepts in caregiver research. *Journal of Nursing Scholarship, 35*, 27–34.

Jones, C., and Shorter-Gooden, K. (2003). *Shifting: The Double Lives of Black Women in America.* New York: Harper Collins.

Kiecolt-Glaser, J., and Newton, T. (2001). Marriage and health: His and hers. *Psychological Bulletin, 127*, 472–503.

Kwong, M.J., Bartholomew, K., Henderson A.J.Z., and Trinke, S.J. (2003). The intergenerational transmission of relationship violence. *Journal of Family Psychology, 17*, 288–301.

Li, L.W. (2005). From caregiving to bereavement: Trajectories of depressive symptoms among wife and daughter caregivers. *Journals of Gerontology: Series B: Psychological Sciences and Social Sciences, 60B*, P190–P198.

Li, L.W., and Seltzer, M.M. (2005). Relationship quality with parent, daughter role salience, and self-esteem of daughter caregivers. *Marriage and Family Review, 37*, 63–82.

Loos, C., and Bowd, A. (1997). Caregivers of persons with Alzheimer's disease: Some neglected implications of the experience of personal loss and grief. *Death Studies, 21*, 501–514.

Lyons, K.S., Zarit, S.H., Sayer, A.G., and Whitlatch, C.J. (2002). Caregiving as a dyadic process: Perspectives from caregiver and receiver. *Journals of Gerontology: Series B: Psychological Sciences and Social Sciences, 57B*, P195–P204.

Mace, N.L., and Rabins, P.V. (2001). *The 36-hour day: A Family Guide to Caring for Persons with Alzheimer's Disease, Related Dementing Illnesses, and Memory Loss in Later Life* (rev. ed.). New York: Warner Books.

Melberg, K. (2005). Family farm transactions in Norway: Unpaid care across three farm generations. *Journal of Comparative Family Studies, 36*, 419–441.

Minkler, M. (2005). American Indian/Alaskan Native grandparents raising grandchildren: Findings from the Census 2000 supplementary survey. *Social Work, 50*, 131–139.

Minkler, M., and Fuller-Thomson, E. (2005). African American grandparents raising grandchildren: A national study using the census 2000 American community survey. *Journals of Gerontology: Series B: Psychological Sciences and Social Sciences, 60B*(2), S82–S92.

Mona, L.R. (2003). Sexual options for people with disabilities: Using personal assistance services for sexual expression. In M.E. Banks and E. Kaschak (Eds.), *Women with Visible and Invisible Disabilities: Multiple Intersections, Multiple Issues, Multiple Therapies* (pp. 211–221). New York: Haworth.

Nabors, N.A., and Pettee, M.F. (2003). Womanist therapy with African American women with disabilities. In M.E. Banks and E. Kaschak (Eds.), *Women with Visible and Invisible Disabilities: Multiple Intersections, Multiple Issues, Multiple Therapies* (pp. 331–341). New York: Haworth Press.

Riggle, E.D.B., Rostosky, S.S., Prather, R.A., and Hamrin, R. (2005). The execution of legal documents by sexual minority individuals. *Psychology, Public Policy, and Law, 11*, 138–163.

Riley, L.D., and Bowen, C. (2005). The sandwich generation: Challenges and coping strategies of multigenerational families. *Family Journal, 13*, 52–58.

Riley-Doucet, C. (2005). Beliefs about the controllability of pain: Congruence between older adults with cancer and their family caregivers. *Journal of Family Nursing, 11*, 225–241.

Rysberg, J.A. (2005). Stress and trauma in the lives of middle-aged and old women. In K. Kendall-Tackett (Ed.), *The Handbook of Women, Stress, and Trauma* (pp. 75–98). New York: Brunner-Routledge.

Sherwood, P.R., Given, C.W., Given, B.A., and von Eye, A. (2005). Caregiver burden and depressive symptoms: Analysis of common outcomes in caregivers of elderly patients. *Journal of Aging and Health, 17*, 125–147.

Simon-Rusinowitz, L., Mahoney, K.J., Loughlin, D.M., and Sadler, M.D. (2005). Paying family caregivers: An effective policy option in the Arkansas Cash and Counseling demonstration and evaluation. *Marriage and Family Review, 37*, 83–105.

Sleath, B., Thorpe, J., Landerman, L.R., Doyle, M., and Clipp, E. (2005). African-American and White caregivers of older adults with dementia: Differences in depressive symptomatology and psychotropic drug use. *Journal of the American Geriatrics Society, 53*, 397–404.

Tatum, B.D. (1999). *Assimilation Blues: Black Families in White Communities—Who Succeeds and Why?* New York: Basic Books.

Terri Schiavo Has Died. (2005, March 31). CNN.com. Retrieved October 17, 2005 from http://www.cnn.com/2005/LAW/03/31/schiavo/.

Tryssenaar, J., and Tremblay, M. (2002). Aging with a serious mental disability in rural northern Ontario: Family members' experiences. *Psychiatric Rehabilitation Journal, 25*, 255–264.

US Census Bureau (2004a). *United States General Demographic Characteristics: 2004*. Retrieved October 12, 2005 from http://factfinder.census.gov/servlet/ADPTable?_bm=y&-geo_id=01000US&-qr_name=ACS_2004_EST_G00_DP1&-ds_name=ACS_2004_EST_G00_&-redoLog=false&-_scrollToRow=104&-format=.

US Census Bureau (2004b). *United States Selected Social Characteristics: 2004*. Retrieved October 12, 2005 from http://factfinder.census.gov/servlet/ADPTable?_bm=y&-qr_name=ACS_2004_EST_G00_DP2&-geo_id=01000US&-ds_name=&-redoLog=false&-format=.

US Department of Health and Human Services, Centers for Disease Control and Prevention, National Center for Health Statistics. (2004a). *NCHS Definitions*. Retrieved May 5, 2006 from http://www.cdc.gov/nchs/datawh/nchsdefs/adl.htm.

US Department of Health and Human Services, Centers for Disease Control and Prevention, National Center for Health Statistics. (2004b). *NCHS Definitions*. Retrieved May 5, 2006 from http://www.cdc.gov/nchs/datawh/nchsdefs/iadl.htm.

Väänänen, A., Buunk, B.P., Kivimäki, M., Pentti, J., and Vahtera, J. (2005). When it is better to give than to receive: Long-term health effects of perceived reciprocity in support exchange. *Journal of Personality and Social Psychology, 89*, 176–193.

Vahtera, J., Kivimäki, M., Väänänen, A., Linna, A., Pentti, J., Helenius H., and Elovainio, M. (2006). Sex differences in health effects of family death or illness: Are women more vulnerable than men? *Psychosomatic Medicine, 68*, 283–291.

Ward-Griffin, C. (2004). Nurses as caregivers of elderly relatives: Negotiating personal and professional boundaries. *Canadian Journal of Nursing Research, 36*, 92–114.

Williams, V., and Robinson, C. (2001). More than one wavelength: Identifying, understanding, and resolving conflicts of interest between people with intellectual disabilities and their family carers. *Journal of Applied Research in Intellectual Disabilities, 14*, 30–46.

Williamson, G.M., Martin-Cook, K., Weiner, M.F., Svetlik, D.A., Saine, K., Hynan, L.S., Dooley, W.K., and Schulz, R. (2005). Caregiver resentment: Explaining why care recipients exhibit problem behavior. *Rehabilitation Psychology, 50*, 215–223.

Winston, C.A. (2003). African American grandmothers parenting AIDS orphans: Concomitant grief and loss. *American Journal of Orthopsychiatry, 73*, 91–100.

Ziemba, R.A., and Lynch-Sauer, J.M. (2005). Preparedness for taking care of elderly parents: "First, you get ready to cry." *Journal of Women & Aging, 17*(1/2), 99–113.

9
Work and Retirement: Challenges and Opportunities for Women Over 50

Judith A. Sugar

> Age puzzles me. I thought it was a quiet time. My seventies were interesting and fairly serene, but my eighties are passionate. I grow more intense as I age.
> Florida Scott-Maxwell (1968), a psychologist, writer, playwright, and suffragist, who began a career in analytical psychology at age 50.

For most people the word *work* conjures up an image of someone employed in a job for which pay is received. Yet, much of the work that women do is unpaid, and, consequently, it is neither recognized nor defined as work. Ignoring women's unpaid labor has detrimental effects on their financial well-being while they are in the labor force and later for their retirement prospects. The psychological, social, and emotional toll of ignoring women's unpaid work is largely unexamined. Furthermore, women face cumulative discrimination in the workplace that begins at their entry into the labor force, continues in their wages and promotions throughout their employment, and then affects their financial resources and benefits in retirement.

Retirement is also an interesting concept for women, because much of the unpaid work that women do continues after they exit from the paid labor force. In fact, the concept of retirement for women has been described as problematic for several reasons, including the fact that women's paid and unpaid work are often interconnected (Onyx & Benton, 1996). In addition, many cannot afford to exit the labor force. Nevertheless, the definition of *retirement* that would fit with most Americans' conceptions early in the new millennium is a period of leisure that follows cessation of a full-time job. Here, too, there is a dearth of studies of women's experiences.

Women live longer than men. It would seem sensible, then, that women should be a major focus of research within the field of aging. As Crose (1997) has pointed out, studying older women's lives has the potential to benefit everyone. Nonetheless, whereas some have argued that research on older women's issues is prolific (e.g., Adams, 1994), others have said that researchers have mostly ignored older women (e.g., Hooyman & Rubinstein, 1997). In the first study to assess those competing claims my colleagues and I (Sugar et al., 2002) surveyed 25 gerontology teaching texts and reference sources published between 1995 and 2001 and more than 1200 journal articles published between 1996 and 2000 in five major gerontology journals. For text and reference sources, the data collected included the number of chapters in which a female-related word was present in the chapter title and the number of pages, according to the index, on which any content on women's issues appeared. For journal articles, the data collected included the number of articles with a female-related word in the title.

The results of the survey were revealing. Most sources had very little content on women's issues at all. Only two gerontology textbooks (of 10 surveyed) and only one gerontology handbook (of 13 surveyed) devoted a chapter to women's issues, and these books also had significantly more pages devoted to those issues than did the textbooks and handbooks with no separate chapters (13.3% versus 4.5%). Thus, it cannot be argued that the latter sources integrated content on women throughout their pages rather than concentrating it in particular chapters. Overall, journals had more content on women, although these numbers were also low; only 241 of 1207 articles (7.5%) focused on women's issues. Among the five journals surveyed, articles on older women's issues were most likely to be published in the *Journals of Gerontology: Medical Sciences* (14.3% of articles) and least likely to be published in the *Journals of Gerontology: Psychological Sciences* (2.5% of articles). There are, of course, excellent sources for scholarship on aging women, including specialty publications such as the *Journal of Women & Aging* and the *Handbook on Women and Aging* (Coyle, 2001). Our focus, however, was on general gerontology textbooks and major reference sources, such as handbooks, because they define the field of gerontology and its central variables (Katz, 2000; McAuley, 2000), and thus, it is critical that their content reflect subject matter that is relevant to women, who are the majority of aging adults. Similarly, journals publish the latest research in a field, and, again, researchers and editors must recognize the importance of studying the aging process of women. Although content on women in middle age was not the focus of the study, there is work on midlife published in gerontology texts and journals. Clearly, the results of the Sugar et al. survey of recent gerontological literature indicate that Hooyman and Rubinstein (1997) were correct that researchers have mostly ignored aging women. Thus, women's aging remains a fertile and important area for future research and publication, which can provide a basis for improved policies and practices that result from it.

Demographic Data on Women in the Workforce and Retired Women

The data available on American women in the workforce, and on retired women, are reported in age categories that do not capture the population of most interest for our purposes in this book. Specifically, employment data are most commonly reported by grouping 25- to 54-year-olds and then 55-year-olds and up, or 65-year-olds and up. Similarly, the youngest age at which retirement data are reported is 55.

TABLE 9.1. Number of women in the United States age 55 years and over by age and race/ethnicity.

Race/ethnicity	Years of age			
	55–64	65–74	75+	Total
White	13,120,000	8,469,000	8,964,000	30,553,000
Black	1,660,000	1,015,000	802,400	3,477,000
Asian	605,000	341,500	278,300	1,224,800
Other[a]	277,000	156,500	96,300	529,800
Total	15,662,000	9,982,000	10,141,000	35,785,000

Note. Adapted from U.S. Census Bureau (2005).
[a] Includes Hispanics/Latinas, American Indians, Native Alaskans, Pacific Islanders, "other" race, and two or more races.

On economic indicators, data are simply not reported separately for 50- to 54-year-olds. Thus, to provide comparable demographic, employment, and retirement data, I have selected the age categories that most closely correspond to our population of interest for this book, namely women 55 years of age or older.

According to the most recent census, there are more than 35 million women 55 years of age or older in the United States (U.S. Census Bureau, 2004). Table 9.1 shows the number of these women by age group and race/ethnicity. Note that there are an additional nine million women in the United States between the ages of 50 and 54.

Career Issues

Cohort differences play a major role in women's career experiences. Since the early years of the women's movement, the number of women in the workforce has increased significantly. Although single women and Black women have always had high rates of participation in the paid workforce, the growth in the numbers of married women, and especially married women with children, has been dramatic. In 1978, 44% of married women with children under age 6 were in the workforce, and by 1998 that percentage had grown to 65% (Costello & Stone, 2001). These cohort differences in the participation of women in the workforce will continue to affect the patterns of employment of female baby boomers and future generations as they age. By their sheer numbers, female workers now have the power to be the architects of a different, and better, workplace environment.

In 2005, almost 11 million women aged 55 and over were employed in the workforce (see Table 9.2), and another 380,000 women were unemployed but looking for work. One pattern of employment evident in Table 9.2 is related to age; specifically, the older women are, the less likely they are to be employed. In fact, consistent across race and ethnicity, most women age 55 or more, who were in the workforce in 2005, were between the ages of 55 and 64. This pattern is due to several factors. One factor is the cohort of today's older women, a majority of whom did not have a history of participating in the paid workforce in their middle-age

TABLE 9.2. Number of women over 55 employed in the workforce in the United States in 2005 by age and race/ethnicity.

Race/ethnicity	Years of age			
	55–64	65–74	75+	Total
White	7,317,000	1,539,000	391,000	7,317,000
Black	844,000	164,000	29,000	1,037,000
Asian	335,000	58,000	16,000	409,000
Other[a]	139,000	35,000	5,000	179,000
Total	8,635,000	1,796,000	441,000	10,872,000

Note. Adapted from U.S. Bureau of Labor Statistics (2005a).
[a] Includes Hispanics/Latinas, American Indians, Native Alaskans, Pacific Islanders, "other" race, and two or more races.

years. Thus, the fact that a large proportion of these women are not employed as they grow older might not be surprising. Other factors that can influence the employment status of older women include their desire to be employed (or not), their health, employers' penchant for hiring them (or not), and the availability of suitable employment where they live. Even though in 2005 most of the employed women in our population of interest were younger than 65, we should note that there were also more than two million women aged 65 or older employed at that same time.

Paid work has several well-recognized meanings, as a source of: income, personal identity (especially in the United States), community status, a sense of accomplishment, and social interaction (Friedmann & Havighurst, 1954). These meanings, as well as much of the research that has followed from them, have been based primarily on the work experiences of White men. The importance of paid work in women's lives has significantly increased over the last half-century, so that many of these meanings are now as relevant to women's lives as they have been to men for some time. On the other hand, women's lives, both in and out of the workforce, are different from men's and consequently lead to different or other meanings of paid work. In addition to being a source of income, financial independence from men has been demonstrated to be an important meaning of labor force participation for many women. This need for independence is sometimes accompanied by concerns about the risks of financial dependence on men or the need for insurance against abandonment or abuse (Altschuler, 2004). The historical lack of opportunities for women to pursue careers in the past and pressures to marry and be a stay-at-home parent have resulted in another meaning of paid work for women—lost dreams and regrets about what might have been. This meaning is often played out by mid- and late-life women going back to school and encouraging and supporting their children, especially their daughters, to pursue an education that will lead to a meaningful career (Altschuler, 2004). With the dramatic shifts in the employment landscape that have already taken place, and many more to come, the issue of the meaning of work will continue to be of interest from research, practical, and policy perspectives.

TABLE 9.3. Sex differences in annual income of full-time workers in the United States: 1970–2004[a].

	1970	1980	1990	2004
Women	$22,918	$25,167	$28,857	$32,101
Men	$38,691	$41,630	$40,612	$41,667
Difference	$15,773	$16,463	$11,755	$9,566
Percentage of difference	41	40	29	23

Note. Adapted from U.S. Census Bureau (2004).
[a] Median income in 2004 dollars.

Salaries and Occupations

The good news about women's salaries in the new millennium is that the longstanding wage gap between women and men has been gradually closing (see Table 9.3). Both the women's movement and its concomitant effects on the increased participation of women in the paid workforce have had their effects on decreasing salary differences between women and men. In 1970, women earned, on average, 40% less than men. By 2004 that gap had been reduced to 23%. The largest reduction occurred between 1980 and 1990 when sex differences in annual income decreased by 11%. The bad news is that women's wages are still significantly lower than men's. And, in 2004 women were still earning less than men earned more than 30 years ago, which reflects the fact that while women's wages have increased, men's wages have remained relatively stagnant over that time period.

Some would argue that the sex differences in salaries are due to differences in women's and men's occupations. As Table 9.4 shows, there are differences in the proportions of female and male workers by occupational type. Women are significantly more likely than are men to be employed in sales and office work and significantly less likely to be employed in production/transportation and natural resources/construction work. (They are equally likely to be employed in management/professional and service work.) Although differences in salaries within occupational types undoubtedly exist, what is clear is that female workers earn less than do male workers in all occupational categories (see Figure 9.1). Sex differences in median salaries range from $2,000 per year for production and

TABLE 9.4. Number and percentage of full-time workers in the United States by occupational type and sex in 2004.

Occupational, category[a]	Total number of workers	Percentage of workers	
		Women	Men
Sales, office	24,950,000	62.3	36.6
Management, professional	36,149,000	50.3	49.7
Service	13,763,000	49.2	50.8
Production, transportation	15,082,000	21.9	78.1
Natural resources, construction	11,280,000	3.9	96.1

Note. Adapted from U.S. Bureau of Labor Statistics (2005b).

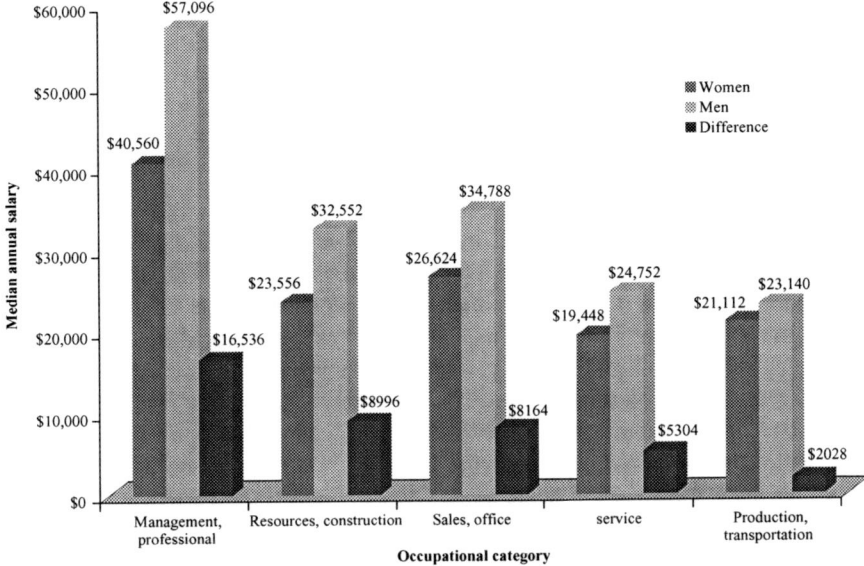

FIGURE 9.1. Sex differences in median annual salaries of American workers in 2004 by occupational categories.

transportation jobs to well over $16,000 per year for management and professional jobs. The two occupational categories where sex differences are the smallest are the two categories with the lowest salaries.

Thus, although some progress has been made in improving women's salaries relative to men's, women are still at a disadvantage in their paychecks. Partly to blame is the lack of mentoring women receive when it comes to negotiating their starting salaries and salary increases. Fortunately, authors are beginning to address this issue by making explicit both the process of salary negotiations and the price of being "nice" (e.g., Babcock & Laschever, 2003; Rose & Danner, 1998), which should help ease this problem for the future.

Over the previous 40 years, women's perseverance in pursuing education to fulfill their career interests has led to greater job opportunities for them. Women now earn more than one-half the bachelor's and master's degrees conferred in the United States (Hussar, 2005). Although they remain the primary holders of traditional women's jobs—women are still most of the registered nurses (93%), dental assistants (98%), elementary school teachers (84%), and librarians (84%)—they have made substantial gains in some professional occupations, at least doubling and even quadrupling their numbers as architects, dentists, physicians, financial managers, and lawyers (Costello & Stone, 2001). They have even made inroads in some well-paid blue-collar occupations traditionally held by men, such as aircraft engine mechanics, truck drivers, police and detectives, and industrial truck and tractor equipment operators (Costello & Stone, 2001). Progress in many occupational arenas, however, has tended to be in entry-level positions rather than senior ones.

Academia is one of those arenas, where women now comprise 45% of Assistant Professors but are still only 24% of full Professors (*Chronicle of Higher Education*, 2006).

Women's Diverse Work Patterns and Career Advancement

Patterns in work history can take a number of forms. The pattern that is often used as the standard or norm is a linear one in which a period of education is followed by a period of work, and then by a period of retirement. This has been the predominant pattern for White men. Many women, on the other hand, take time away from employment during their careers, primarily to give birth to or adopt children and to care for their young children or for their older or ill relatives. Until recently, the biggest family issue for female baby boomers was childcare—its availability and affordability, and how to "balance" paid employment and childcare responsibilities. Increases in longevity, however, have introduced a new family issue that may overtake childcare as the greatest challenge to women's lives—parentcare.

Baby boomers comprise the first generation in American history to have more parents than children. They are also the first generation that is likely to spend more years caring for their parents than for their children (Dychtwald, 1999). In fact, female baby boomers may spend 20 or 30 years caring for their parents, in contrast to 18 years caring for their children. And women—mothers, daughters, daughters-in-law, aunts, and grandmothers—are overwhelmingly the caregivers of both the older and the younger generations (Stone et al., 1987). The fact that as they reach middle age many women find themselves in the middle of dealing with both childcare and parentcare has led to them being called the "sandwich generation." See Chapter 8 for a discussion of how caregiving affects midlife women's lives.

The effects of childcare considerations on mothers who work outside the home have been documented for many years. Little research, though, has been conducted on the extent to which taking time off from full-time employment to care for older relatives has impacted women's income, career advancement, or both. Caregiving responsibilities of any kind often lead women to cut back their work hours, to rearrange their work schedules, or to change jobs so that they can have greater flexibility to accommodate caregiving work. When women are younger, childcare may lead them to leave the workforce for a period of time. As we are only beginning to learn how, when women are older, caregiving for their parents, parents-in-law, or other relatives may lead them to decline promotions, change jobs, or take early retirement.

Full-time versus Part-time Work

One of the main reasons women today work part-time rather than full-time is to enable them to fulfill caregiving responsibilities for family members. Although more American women at all ages are employed full-time than part-time (52 versus 18 million), women are much less likely to be full-time workers and much more

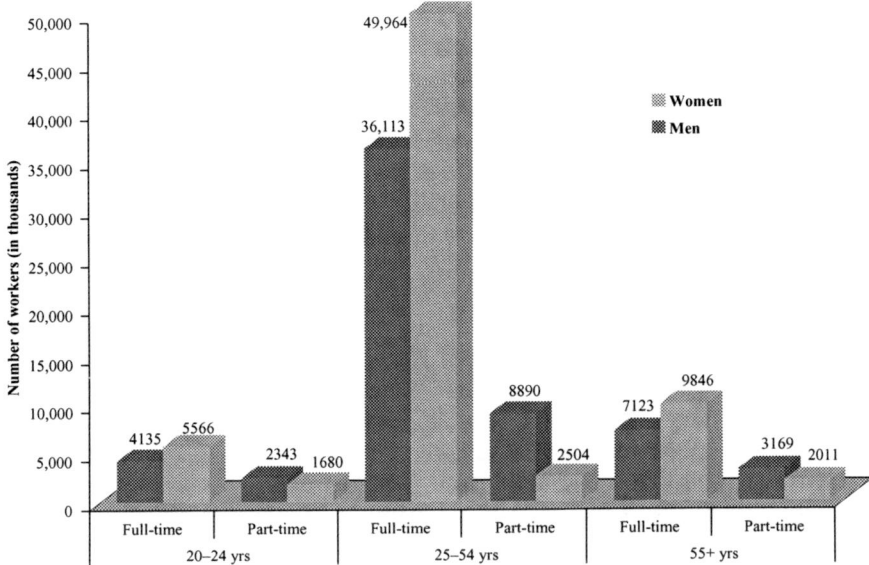

FIGURE 9.2. Number of full-time and part-time American workers in 2004 by age and sex.

likely to be part-time workers than are men. In fact, during the critical years between 25 and 54 years of age, when employees are in the growth years of their careers for earnings, promotions, and accumulating retirement savings, only 80% of employed women are working full-time compared to 95% of men (see Figure 9.2). Of course, part-time employees are also less likely to have the employment income to invest and to save for retirement, and they are less likely to be promoted because part-time jobs seldom lead to promotions. Working part-time, as opposed to full-time, leads to at least two additional problems for women as they age: The amount they will contribute toward social security and other retirement vehicles will be less than if they were full-time workers, and they are less likely than they would be as full-time workers to receive benefits, especially health care and employers' pension contributions.

Income and Career Advancement

Recently, a survey of a nationally representative group of more than 2400 women with degrees in higher education was conducted to learn more about what has been termed the "opt-out revolution"—an apparent trend of today's professional women to drop out of the full-time workforce, reputedly permanently (Hewlett & Luce, 2005). Among other questions, the women were asked about their experiences on returning to their jobs after taking leaves for various periods of time. The effect on their salaries was striking: Compared to women who had not taken time out, those who took leaves of 1 year or less lost an average of 11% in their salaries, and those who took leaves of 3 years or more lost an average of 37% in their salaries. They were also significantly less likely to receive promotions after their return to work.

The Hewlett and Luce study also debunked the claim by recent media reports that a new generation of young women is giving up their careers to return to the traditional role of housewife for the long haul. For many women, of course, taking a hiatus in the midst of their working lives to devote time to their family is not a realistic option. Even for professional women who take that hiatus, however, most (93%) were clear that they wanted to, or planned to, return to their careers.

Retirement Issues

Most of the available demographic data on American retirees can be found through reports based on social security benefits. These numbers are reasonably good approximations for male retirees because the vast majority of male employees in the United States are eligible for Social Security benefits at age 62. However, these numbers are poor approximations for the current cohort of female retirees over age 50 because many of those women do not qualify for their own social security benefits, and the available data do not distinguish between women's own benefits from their employment and the benefits to which they are entitled as widows. Currently, accurate data on the numbers of female retirees over age 50 are impossible to come by. The best demographic data available, which are on women not in the workforce, are presented in Table 9.5.

According to the U.S. Bureau of Labor Statistics (2005a), more than 24 million women age 55 or older were not in the workforce in 2005. Similar to the workforce data reported in Table 9.2, more women were out of the workforce after age 64 than at younger ages, except for the category of "other" (which includes Hispanics/Latinas, American Indians, Native Alaskans, Pacific Islanders, "other" race, and two or more races). A major reason that the numbers do not continue to increase for Women of Color is that their lifespans are currently shorter than those of White women.

TABLE 9.5. Number of women over 55 *not* in the workforce in the United States in 2005 by age and race/ethnicity.

Race/ethnicity	Years of age			
	55–64	65–74	75+	Total
White	5,578000	6,878,000	8,562,000	21,018,000
Black	769,000	839,000	773,000	2,381,000
Asian	250,000	281,000	262,000	793,000
Other[a]	131,000	119,000	91,000	341,000
Total	6,728,000	8,117,000	9,688,000	24,533,000

Note. Adapted from U.S. Bureau of Labor Statistics (2005b).
[a] Includes Hispanics/Latinas, American Indians, Native Alaskans, Pacific Islanders, "other" race, and two or more races.

Although age 65 is often thought of as the "traditional" age of retirement, the idea of retirement as a tradition is paradoxical. Retirement is a relatively new phenomenon; it began in the mid-twentieth century, and occurs primarily in Western, industrialized countries. And, many Americans have yet to experience it because their jobs have not provided them with adequate retirement pensions. For women, in addition to the problem of inadequate pensions, even if they retire from full-time jobs, they rarely retire from their "second shifts" of domestic work and family caregiving responsibilities.

Policies That Affect Women's Retirement

Of all the policies adopted in the United States during the twentieth century that have affected retirement, social security has had the greatest impact. Enacted in 1935, social security was always intended to provide a safety net for American workers in their elder years (Roosevelt, 1935), but for many it has been far more than that. In fact, social security represents more than 80% of the income of older adults in the lowest two quintiles of earnings (U.S. Census Bureau, 2002). Furthermore, although most Americans regard social security as valuable only for older adults, it actually benefits Americans of all ages because it removes older people from the workforce, thus freeing up jobs for younger people, and it often obviates the necessity for family members to take care of their elders, thereby freeing up their time and resources for other pursuits.

For most American workers, mandatory retirement became obsolete in 1978 with the passage of the Age Discrimination in Employment Act (ADEA). As of January 1994, one of the last bastions of mandatory retirement was abolished when university and college faculty members were no longer required to retire at age 70. Thus, with the exception of a handful of occupations for which it is deemed unsafe to have older workers (e.g., airline pilots, police, firefighters), employees are no longer required to leave their jobs when they reach a particular age. It is interesting that, subsequent to ADEA, retirement at earlier and earlier ages actually became more common, and only recently has the retirement age begun to rise again slightly. During the 1980s and 1990s, in the wake of corporate mergers and downsizing, informal pressures and new incentives to retire replaced mandatory retirement as a way to remove midlife and older adults from the workforce (Robertson, 2000).

Changes to a number of policies and practices will affect retirement prospects for women in the twenty-first century. One of these changes is the removal of the earnings penalty from social security. Prior to 1997, retirees lost a substantial proportion of their annual social security benefits if they chose to continue working. With the amendments to the Social Security Act in 1997 and 2002, new cohorts of retirees will be able to earn sizeable annual incomes to supplement Social Security benefits without financial penalty (up to $30,000 in 2002, to be subsequently indexed to wage growth). Another change that will impact the retirement prospects for future cohorts of retirees has been the move by the private sector from defined-benefit to defined-contribution retirement plans.

Defined-Benefit and Defined-Contribution Retirement Plans

Defined-benefit retirement plans are those in which retirees' annual pensions are based on the salaries they earn while they are employed and their years of service with the employer. In this type of plan, what is defined is the level of pension income that will be achieved by the employees upon their retirement. The less orderly careers of women put them at a disadvantage in these plans because benefits depend upon a minimum number of years of work for the same employer.

Defined-contribution retirement plans, on the other hand, are those in which an employer deposits a specified percentage of an employee's annual salary into his or her individual tax-deferred pension fund, and this percentage is usually matched by the employee. In this type of plan, what is defined is the amount that the employer will contribute toward an employee's pension, not what the employee who retires will receive as income from that pension. Although these plans are portable (i.e., do not depend on staying with the same employer), the pension income from this type of plan depends on the employee's decisions about how to invest the contributions among the available options and on the vagaries of the national economy that affect those investments (e.g., inflation, interest rates, stock market growth). The private sector is increasingly shifting the burden of risk for pension plans to employees by replacing defined-benefit plans with defined-contribution plans. From 1985 to 1998, the number of defined-benefit plans decreased by 67%, whereas the number of defined-contribution plans increased by 46% (American Benefits Council, 2004). Furthermore, unlike defined-benefit pensions, defined-contribution pensions are not insured by the Employee Retirement Income Security Act (ERISA). Thus, the dual guarantees of known levels of retirement income that were available to earlier retirees through defined-benefits plans will not exist for most future retirees.

Poverty and Women's Longevity

One of the saddest commentaries on our society is that so many women live in poverty during their elder years. The gerontology literature attributes much of older women's poverty to their longevity; the claim is that because women live for more years than men, they are more likely than are men to outlive their financial resources. Although it is certainly true that, on average, women live longer than do men, it seems more than disingenuous to blame older women's poverty on their longevity. In fact, discriminatory policies and practices in our society result in women beginning retirement age with substantially fewer financial resources than do men because most of the income and benefits for older Americans are based on a model of White men's full-time and long-term employment in the workforce. Retirement policies effectively penalize women who work part-time or who take time out to raise families and to provide care for elderly family members. What makes matters worse is the consistently lower salaries that women earn in the workplace.

To get a sense of just how much lower a woman's earnings would be over her lifetime of work, I took the hypothetical case of Sarah who began full-time employment in 1975 and wanted to retire in 2015. I used the average sex differences in salary in 1970, 1980, 1990, and 2004 to interpolate and sum the annual salary shortfalls for Sarah during her 40 years of full-time paid work. The resulting total shortfall was a whopping $480,000. This amount does not include the interest or potential additional income that would accrue with the investment of the "extra" annual salary that Sarah would have earned if she had been a male employee. Furthermore, both her social security earnings and private pension (if she has one) are also affected by her lower income because they are both based on employment earnings. And, because employers often match employees' contributions to private pension plans, Sarah's employer would also contribute significantly fewer dollars to her pension savings than would be the case had her salary been higher. Conservatively, we can estimate that the net effect of Sarah's lower income would be that she would end up with at least $1,000,000 less at retirement than her male counterpart would have. That amount for every retired woman would go a long way toward ending poverty among older women.

The Future of Retirement for Women

Middle-aged women of today blazed a new trail for women in the workplace and, although all hopes for that frontier have not yet been realized, there have been significant achievements. These same women will once again blaze a new trail—this time creating models for what women can do in retirement. There are certainly challenges ahead for women in retirement, but there are also new opportunities to define the very meaning and structure of it. Women's own labor force participation, accompanied by various legislative actions (to improve pension rights, for example), has given them much more independence than previous generations of women have had. Many of them will have the latitude to choose among numerous options, from pursuing new careers (Brontë, 1995), to engaging in popular leisure activities such as travel, to spending more time with friends and family, to getting involved in politics.

There is also the potential for continued earnings in retirement without the financial penalties on social security income that occurred in the past. This same potential, though, in conjunction with the likelihood that future private pensions will depend more heavily on employees' investment prowess with their defined contributions, will likely lead to greater expectations that older Americans will fend for themselves in retirement. A concomitant outcome may be a diminishing interest in ensuring that social security continues to act as a safety net for America's aging citizens. In addition, rapidly increasing costs of health care, reductions in employers' health care benefits for retirees, and the uneasy future of Medicare together may lead most Americans to decide that they will likely have to forgo retirement to ensure that they will be able to maintain a reasonable quality of life in their elder years.

The idea of retirement often conjures up an image of retirees engaged in leisure activities. This image may have been a good picture of retirement for many workers in the past. In 1996, for example, only 17% of women and 27% of men between

TABLE 9.6. Personal definitions of retirement of American pre-retirees aged 50–70.

Possible aspects of retirement	Percentage of respondents[a]
Spending more time with family and friends	78
A chance to relax	73
A chance to have more fun	73
A chance to do things you never had time for	72
Receiving retirement benefits from social security or pension payments	72
A chance to travel	67
Doing volunteer or charity work	57
Slowing down and working fewer hours	56
Working for enjoyment, not money	53
A chance to stop working for pay completely	48
Having to do some kind of work to help pay bills	42
A chance to leave your main career to try a different type of work	28
Feeling less useful or less productive	20

Note. Adapted from AARP (2003a), p. 13.

[a] For each possible aspect, the percentage is based on those respondents ($N = 1637$) who indicated it was very much or somewhat part of their personal definition of retirement.

65 and 69 years of age, were participating in the workforce (Purcell, 2000). However, evidence is accumulating that retirement will be quite different for the baby boomer cohort. Based on a nationwide survey of 2001 employees between 50 and 70 years of age, AARP (2003a) reported that 63% of preretirees planned to work *at least* part-time after the age of 65, and another 5% said that they planned never to retire. These preretirees' personal definitions of retirement in part reflect the new financial realities for this and future cohorts of retirees. Their definitions also reflect different attitudes toward work. Table 9.6 lists the proportion of survey respondents who indicated that specific aspects of retirement were "very much" or "somewhat" part of their personal definition of retirement. Many of their choices are related to postretirement work, including "slowing down and working fewer hours," "having to do some kind of work to help pay bills," and "a chance to leave your main career to try a different type of work." Nevertheless, middle-aged Americans are looking forward to many aspects of retirement enjoyed by current retirees, including spending more time with family and friends, relaxing, having more fun, and "doing things they have never had time for."

Similarly, the reasons given by Americans age 50 and over for working in retirement are diverse. When they are forced to choose only one, financial concerns are paramount, but most Americans have other reasons, too, which include a desire to be mentally and physically active, generativity, pleasure, and social interaction (AARP, 2005a; see Table 9.7).

A vast array of volunteer and recreational choices already exist, and many more can be expected as the marketplace more fully recognizes the potential for retirees to be engaged in their communities and to seek new experiences. In 2002 Americans age 55 and older contributed more than $160 billion to society through their volunteer and caregiving activities (Johnson & Schaner, 2005). Furthermore,

TABLE 9.7. Major reasons given by older Americans for working in retirement.

Reasons	Percentage of respondents[a]
Financial	
Income	61
Health benefits	52
Cognitive	
Staying mentally alert	54
Learning new things	17
Physical	
Staying physically active	49
Generativity	
Remaining productive/useful	47
Helping others	29
Pleasure	
Enjoying fun activities	37
Pursuing a dream	14
Social	
Being around others	24

Note. Adapted from AARP (2005a, March).
[a] For each reason, the numbers are the percent of respondents who indicated that it was important to them.

initiatives such as the Gerontological Society of America's research on *Civic Engagement in an Older America* to increase older adults' opportunities for civic and social engagement, and the alliance between AARP and *Monster*, a leading online career site, to provide career resources including local job listings (AARP, 2005b) are only the beginning of what will be many exciting new possibilities for the work and retirement of women over 50.

Recommendations for Research and Policy on Work and Retirement

A significant portion of the more recent research on work and retirement issues of adults over age 50 has been conducted by AARP (e.g., AARP, 2002, 2003a, 2003b, 2005a). That AARP would have a major interest in these issues in this population is understandable because its target market is the American population age 50 and over. Nevertheless, it is disappointing that its reports have so little information regarding women per se. AARP's reports include isolated examples of sex differences for some measures, but analyses of the data it collects from female respondents are conspicuously absent. In its report on *Boomers at Midlife* (AARP, 2003b), for example, of the 96 tables of data, only nine show women's responses, and of the 16 tables of data dedicated to race/ethnicity, none show women's responses separately.

When it comes to retirement issues, it may be somewhat less surprising that the vast majority of research focuses on retirees or soon-to-be retirees who are male. Retirement is usually defined as cessation of a full-time job, and, until recently, most women have not been employed full-time for long enough to be said to retire or to qualify for their own social security benefits. Furthermore, researchers have not wanted to deal with the complexity of women's multiple entries and exits from the workforce and their attendant implications for retirement.

In addition to focusing on men, retirement research has also focused heavily on the financial issues of leaving the full-time workforce—financial planning for retirement, methods of accumulating wealth, and managing assets after retirement—and has largely ignored the social, emotional, and psychological issues. Employers, too, when they offer seminars or workshops on retirement for their employees, typically devote the time to the financial issues.

There is a substantial body of literature on women's careers and work experiences, but there are still too few data in this arena, and with the rapidly changing work environment much of what we know needs to be reconceptualized or completely overhauled (Moen & Roehling, 2005). We also have much to learn about women's retirement, notwithstanding more recent publications (e.g., Hall, 2002; Mellor & Rehr, 2005; Riggs, 2004). More research is needed on issues related to retirement for women. Attention should be paid to the diversity among women, including race/ethnicity, sexuality, ability status, and partner and parental status. Even basic demographic data are needed. Topics that are underexplored, or not explored at all, include decision-making about retirement, activities and work after retirement; and psychological effects of work, work past the "traditional" age of retirement, and retirement, including how they impact personal identity, self-esteem, and social well-being.

Women who pioneered working full-time are now pioneering the stage of life beyond full-time employment. There are few role models. Many women are disappointed and frustrated that, after so many years of fighting for equal rights in the workplace, there could still be such large gaps in wages and benefits, as well as employment and retirement policies that still adversely affect women. The wage gaps are bad enough in and of themselves, but they also have long-term and significant consequences for women's quality of life as they age.

Policy issues to be addressed include current and proposed provisions of social security and amendments to the Social Security Act to overcome its inherent discrimination against women. Changes to social security should include eliminating the possibility that partners can opt out of survivor coverage and allowing adjustments for interruptions in work histories that are a consequence of childcare and parentcare. With lower salaries throughout their careers, women are significantly more likely than are men to become impoverished as they age, so improving salaries for women should also be a priority. Such changes, of course, will have positive impacts not just for women, but for everyone.

Rethinking Work and Retirement

In place of a linear life pattern of education, followed by work, followed by retirement, a cyclic life pattern seems to be more suitable and attractive, especially given the increasing longevity of both women and men. A cyclic life pattern is one in which education, work, and leisure are intermingled. Thus, for example, a period of education could be followed by work, then more education, then some leisure, then more work, then leisure again, etc.

Linear life pattern

| education | work | retirement/leisure |

Cyclic life pattern

| education | work | education | leisure | work | leisure | education |

This idea, of course, is not new to American women, and, in fact, has been quite common for many of them. What is new, though, is to use the cyclic pattern as a model for education, work, and leisure across the lifespan and to develop policies and practices that would support it. In addition, it would advantageous to expand and create new opportunities for work other than full-time "permanent" jobs. Limited time, part-time, and project-oriented jobs that are meaningful and fulfilling would be desirable to many people. Women of all ages would benefit from these new choices if they were supported in the public and private spheres and if they improved the quality of life in work and retirement.

We need to rethink the work environment and develop new policies and practices to make room for the millions of middle-aged women and men who do not want to exit completely and permanently from the workforce when they reach the age where they could begin to collect social security, private pensions, or both. To provide the opportunities most future older adults desire will require reshaping jobs as well as the workplace to accommodate part-time employees of all kinds—those who would like to work full-time for a few days a week, those who would like to work for a few hours every weekday, perhaps sharing a job, those who would like to work on time-limited projects perhaps full-time for a few months each year, and so forth. With unprecedented numbers of women poised for retirement, the future for "midcourse" women (Moen, 2003) with unprecedented numbers of healthy years of life before them is wide open.

Aging is not 'lost youth' but a new stage of opportunity and strength.

Betty Friedan (1994)

Acknowledgments. Preparation of this chapter was supported in part by the Gerontology Academic Program at the University of Nevada, Reno. The author wishes to thank Courtney Benvenuto, Susan G. Harris, and Erik Schwinger for research assistance.

References

AARP. (2002). *Staying Ahead of the Curve: The AARP Work and Career Study*. Washington, DC: Author.

AARP. (2003a). *Staying Ahead of the Curve 2003: The AARP Working in Retirement Study*. Washington, DC: Author.

AARP. (2003b). *Boomers at Midlife. The AARP Life Stage Study, Wave 2.* Washington, DC: Author.

AARP. (2005a, March). *Attitudes of Individuals 50 and Older Toward Phased Retirement.* Online poll of 2,167 workers over 50. Retrieved March, 2006 from http://www.aarp.org.

AARP. (2005b, May 23). *Monster and AARP Announce Alliance to Help 50+ Workers.* Retrieved February, 2006 from http://www.aarp.org.

Adams, R.G. (1994). Older men's friendship patterns. In E.H. Thompson, Jr. (Ed.), *Older Men's Lives* (pp. 159–177). Thousand Oaks, CA: Sage.

Altschuler, J. (2004). Beyond money and survival: The meaning of paid work among older women. *International Journal of Aging and Human Development, 58,* 223–239.

American Benefits Council. (2004). *Pensions at the Precipice: The Multiple Threats Facing Our Nation's Defined Benefit Pension System.* Washington, DC: Author. Available at http://www.americanbenefitscouncil.org.

Babcock, L., and Laschever, S. (2003). *Women Don't Ask: Negotiation and the Gender Divide.* Princeton, NJ: Princeton University Press.

Brontë, L. (1995). *The Longevity Factor: The New Reality of Long Careers and how it Can Lead to Richer Lives.* New York: HarperCollins.

Chronicle of Higher Education. (2006, August 26). Almanac issue 2005–6.

Costello, C.B., and Stone, A.J. (Eds.). (2001). *The American Woman 2001–2002: Getting to the Top.* New York: Norton.

Coyle, J.M. (Ed.). (2001). *Handbook on Women and Aging.* Westport, CT: Praeger.

Crose, R. (1997). *Why Women Live Longer than Men... and What Men Can Learn from Them.* San Francisco: Jossey-Bass.

Dychtwald, K. (1999). *Age Power: How the 21st Century Will Be Ruled by the New Old.* New York: Penguin Putnam.

Friedan, B. (1994, March 20). Quoted in *Parade Magazine.* Retrieved May 2006 from http://womenshistory.about.com/od/quotes/a/betty_friedan.htm.

Friedmann, E., and Havighurst, R.I. (1954). *The Meaning of Work and Retirement.* Chicago, IL: University of Chicago Press.

Hall, P. (2002). *The Bonus Years: Women and Retirement.* New York: Miranda Press.

Hewlett, S.A., and Luce, C.B. (2005, March). Off-ramps and on-ramps. Keeping talented women on the road to success. *Harvard Business Review,* pp. 43–54.

Hooyman, N.R., and Rubinstein, R.L. (1997). Is aging more problematic for women than men? In A.E. Scharlach and L.W. Kaye (Eds.), *Controversial Issues in Aging* (pp. 125–135). Boston: Allyn & Bacon.

Hussar, W.J. (2005). *Projections of Education Statistics to 2014* (NCES 2005-074). U.S. Department of Education, National Center for Education Statistics. Washington, DC: U.S. Government Printing Office. Available through http://nces.ed.gov.

Johnson, R.W., and Schaner, S.G. (2005, September). Value of unpaid activities by older Americans tops $160 billion per year. *Perspectives on Productive Aging,* Number 4. Washington, DC: Urban Institute. Available at http://www.urban.org.

Katz, S. (2000). Reflections on the gerontological handbook. In T.R. Cole, R. Kastenbaum, and R.E. Ray (Eds.), *Handbook for the Humanities and Aging* (2nd ed., pp. 405–418). New York: Springer.

McAuley, W.J. (2000). Defining the field of gerontology through introductory texts. *Gerontologist, 40,* 242–246.

Mellor, M.J., and Rehr, H. (Eds.). (2005). *Baby Boomers. Can My Eighties Be Like my Fifties?* New York: Springer.

Moen, P. (2003). Midcourse. Reconfiguring careers and community service for a new life stage. *Contemporary Gerontology, 9*, 87–94.

Moen, P., and Roehling, P. (2005). *The Career Mystique: Cracks in the American Dream.* Lanham, MD: Rowan & Littlefield.

Onyx, J., and Benton, P. (1996). Retirement: A problematic concept for older women. *Journal of Women and Aging, 8*, 19–35.

Purcell, P.J. (2000, October). Older workers: Employment and retirement trends. *Monthly Labor Review*, pp. 19–30.

Riggs, K.E. (2004). *Granny@work: Aging and New Technology on the Job in America.* New York: Routledge.

Robertson, A. (2000). "I saw the handwriting on the wall": Shades of meaning in reasons for early retirement. *Journal of Aging Studies, 14*, 63–79.

Roosevelt, F.D. (1935, August 14). *Presidential Statement on Signing the Social Security Act.* Available at www.ssa.gov/history/fdrstmts.html.

Rose, S., and Danner, M.J. (1998). Money matters: The art of negotiation for women faculty. In L.H. Collins, J.C. Chrisler, and K. Quina (Eds.), *Arming Athena: Career Strategies for Women in Academe* (pp. 157–186). Thousand Oaks, CA: Sage.

Scott-Maxwell, F. (1968). *The Measure of My Days.* New York: Knopf.

Stone, R., Cafferata, G.L., and Sangl, J. (1987). Caregivers of the frail elderly: A national profile. *Gerontologist, 27*, 616–626.

Sugar, J.A., Anstee, J.L.K., Desrochers, S., and Jambor, E.E. (2002). Gender biases in gerontological education: The status of older women. *Gerontology & Geriatrics Education, 22*, 43–53.

U.S. Bureau of Labor Statistics. (2005a). *Employment Status of the Civilian Noninstitutional Population by Age, Sex, and Race. [Household data Table 3].* Available at http://www.bls.gov/cps.

U.S. Bureau of Labor Statistics. (2005b). *Women in the Labor Force: A Databook. [Table 18. Median usual weekly earnings of full-time wage and salary workers by detailed occupation and sex, 2004 annual averages].* Available at http://www.bls.gov/cps/wlf-databook2005.htm.

U.S. Census Bureau. (2002). *Current Population Survey. Annual Social and Economic Supplement.* Available at http://factfinder.census.gov.

U.S. Census Bureau. (2004). *Current Population Survey. Annual Social and Economic Supplement.* Available at http://factfinder.census.gov.

U.S. Census Bureau. (2005). *Annual Estimates of the Population by Age and Sex for the United States.* Available at http://factfinder.census.gov.

10
Empowerment: A Prime Time for Women Over 50

Florence L. Denmark and Maria D. Klara

In preparing this chapter, the first author noted: "As someone who achieved a variety of offices and received many awards after age 50, I felt very much in control of my own life, but in no way felt that I was able to or wanted to control others." Thus, although it is important to understand that empowerment and power are tightly intertwined, these two concepts are different.

Power is often related to our ability to make others do what we want, regardless of their own wishes or interests. For most people, the word "power" typically brings to mind thoughts concerning control and domination (Page & Czuba, 1999). Traditional social science emphasizes power as influence and control, often treating power as a commodity or structure separate from human action. In this way, power can be viewed as unchanging or unchangeable, and available only to a select few (Page & Czuba, 1999).

Alternatively, empowerment refers to individuals gaining command over their own destinies (*American Heritage Dictionary*, 2000) as well as helping others to attain this control as well. Something that is empowering makes individuals feel more confident that they are in control of their own lives. Empowerment involves learning to redefine who we are and what we can do, to speak in our own voice, and to change the way we perceive our relationships to institutionalized power (Chamberlin, 1997). In general, an individual or even a group moves from a state of relative powerlessness to power through the empowerment process (Pillai, 1995). This process encompasses attitudes, values, and beliefs about the self, especially beliefs about the ability to exert control over one's destiny (Chadiha et al., 2004).

Empowering others is the process of supporting people to construct new meanings and use their freedom to choose new ways to respond to the world, often to the benefit of others. Empowering others involves providing individuals with the appropriate tools and resources to enhance their self-confidence and self-esteem, to develop leadership skills, and to strive for personal and professional success. Empowering others entails making a systematic and sustained effort to provide others with more information, knowledge, support, and opportunities to use their power for mutual benefit.

Yoder and Kahn (1992) suggested a reconceptualization of power; in this perspective, empowerment can be viewed as the *power-to*, rather than *power-over*. Power-over refers to the coercion and domination of one group over another group, or one person over another person. This power structure can be seen in societal, organizational, interpersonal, and individual levels, and it is used to force a person or entity to do what one individual wants. On the other hand, *power-to* equates to personal empowerment. In this conceptualization, individuals have the power to control their own feelings, thoughts, and actions. The focus is not on controlling others, but rather on using personal power to make improvements in one's life and to gain success for oneself. The *power-to* approach views empowerment as more of a process than an entity; the focus is on power as energy, potential, and competence, as opposed to domination, coercion, and/or competition (Browne, 1995). Such an assessment of power considers the empowerment of women and men to include women and men not only empowering themselves (i.e., developing personal agency) but also changing broader social structures (i.e., collective activism). According to Browne (1995), this form of empowerment is a process of liberation of self and others; it is a life force, a potential, a capacity, a form of growth and energy, where one works toward building both community and connection to others rather than solely striving toward achievement for one's individual good. This definition indicates that power is much more than coercion and domination; it is relational, is sustained by societal forces, and is a dynamic process (Yoder, 2003).

Empowerment may also be viewed as a primary goal of feminist therapy, and the process begins with the assumption that the therapist and the client are equal in the therapy dyad (Denmark et al., 2005). Although clinical and counseling psychologists view personal empowerment (i.e., agency) as a step toward enhanced psychological well-being, feminist psychologists integrate both individualistic independence and communal interdependence into their conceptions. Feminist psychologists found the traditional psychological notion of power, with its emphasis on dominance, control, or influence over others, discomforting, and they emphasize that power must be understood as relational. Thus, power exists within the context of a relationship between people or things; it does not exist in isolation, nor is it inherent in individuals (Page & Czuba, 1999). Thus, along these lines, women feel empowered in and by themselves and in their relationships (Yoder, 2003).

This chapter covers issues related to empowerment, including how feminist psychologists view empowerment; the effects of culture, race, and class on empowerment; how women can help other women become empowered; the role of women's organizations; and international policies that promote the empowerment of women. Empowerment is also discussed in terms of midlife and how growing older affects women's sense of empowerment during different phases of their lives. Feminist women were asked to comment on their views of empowerment, and their perspectives are used to help us to illustrate this concept.

Feminist Women Look at Empowerment

To discover how feminist psychologists view empowerment, a questionnaire was distributed to 100 feminist women, 25 of whom responded. The majority reported that they believe that women are most empowered during midlife, between the ages of 40 and 60. In contrast, for men, the respondents indicated a much wider range: Men are most empowered between the ages of 30 and 70. The respondents indicated that women were the least empowered below the age of 30 and above the age of 70, and the majority identified 80 and older as the least empowered age group for men. This perception of a gender difference is noteworthy. The age span of empowerment for men is perceived as twice as great as that of women, and the least empowered men are seen as 10 years older than the least empowered women.

How Can We Increase Empowerment for Women?

In addition to gender, other factors related to empowerment that respondents reported as most important were: education, occupation, socioeconomic status, holding political office, organizational activities, and ethnicity. Answers to this question were varied, and yet all pointed to the importance of empowerment in various spheres of women's lives. The following are some of the suggestions respondents gave for increasing women's empowerment.

First, many respondents spoke about the need for empowerment in the political system. Through this empowerment, women can become more organized collectively and, thereby, influence important social issues. In this sense, empowerment is characterized as an active entity: It involves fighting for good legislation, involving oneself in all aspects of society, influencing legislators, as well as communicating one's ideas and attitudes. In this view of activism, many of the respondents spoke about the necessity to involve the younger generation and to teach that through an active, empowered stance, change can be made. Individuals in high positions should use their influence in order to empower others and to push for social changes that will result in the equality of all people. Therefore, the relationship between empowerment and change was stated repeatedly in responses from the participants.

A second premise that ran through many responses was encouragement and the belief that this was a necessary activity for further empowerment. Respondents believed that women first need to acknowledge that they have the right to be empowered. In other words, empowerment encourages women to view themselves as centers of power, teaches them how to use that power, and instructs them in how to believe that they can accomplish the things that they wish to do.

Another common theme that ran through the respondents' suggestions was the significance of education for both women and men. Women and men should not be positioned against each other, but rather both should be encouraged to use their resources for the benefit of all. Some believed that mutuality is the goal for all people; therefore, empowerment is not meant to be an "us against them" mentality. Education for both women and men was seen as critical to foster empowerment. According to Lips (2005), making gender stereotypes less rigid should be empowering for both women and men, as it increases their sense of effectiveness and self-actualization. Many of the respondents reported that they believe it is important that individuals organize and work together for mutual empowerment.

As noted by the respondents, midlife is often deemed the age period during which women are most empowered. It is the time when women realize that they have accomplished a great deal in their lives and that they have the education and knowledge of the world needed to advocate successfully for themselves and others. Many women in midlife have taken on leadership roles and are in positions of power and leadership, which helps them to advocate successfully for themselves (thus empowering themselves) and also to aid in the empowerment of others (Babladelis, 1999).

Midlife, Aging, and Empowerment

It is helpful to understand the political, economic, cultural, and societal situation in which women find themselves during midlife. In U.S. society, older women, despite often leading rewarding and productive lives, fall prey to negative stereotypes. Women in midlife and beyond are typically viewed as grey, wrinkled, and no longer sexually attractive. They are often excluded from social situations and undervalued by employers. Aging is something that is embarrassingly covered up—grey hair is often dyed and saggy faces are often surgically lifted. Television often shows older women taking aspirin, Geritol, and baking sweets for their grandchildren (Lott, 1987). Women in this age group are frequently depicted as stubborn, helpless, forgetful, and dependent—if they are shown on television at all.

Aging in Western societies has often been associated with issues related to declining health, social care, and welfare. These issues have dominated the study of aging, which has caused exceedingly negative accounts of later life. By assuming that fulfillment in aging is dependent on the ability of individuals to accept or adapt to physical and social change, we are perpetuating the stereotype of aging as a period of inevitable decline or loss and something to be endured. Too much emphasis is placed on personality and physiological adjustment and not enough on social inequalities that begin in midlife (Wray, 2004).

On a positive note, although many individuals view midlife development for women in a pessimistic manner, others realize that change is possible for women during this developmental period. For the majority of women, midlife is not characterized by a deterioration of capacities, but rather the opposite—it is a time of productivity and happiness (Denmark et al., 2005). Many women over 50 are in the prime of their lives, able to negotiate successfully many spheres of life including home, family, career, and friends. Those who view midlife as a time of productivity focus on the potential of women during midlife for increased competence and a greater sense of identity, which is the essence of empowerment (Stewart et al., 2001).

Development Stage: Midlife

Identity is typically viewed as an achievement of adolescence or early adulthood; however, some psychologists, particularly Erikson, have suggested that women and men might not achieve their identities at the same point in development. Rather, Erikson proposed that women might not achieve a sense of identity until later in life, in the context of intimate relationships. Identity development seems to have important implications for well-being in midlife. For instance, research has indicated that identity development is positively related to midlife self-esteem and life satisfaction in women (Stewart et al., 2001).

Erikson's theory also posits that midlife adults face the conflict of "generativity versus stagnation" and acquire the ego strength (i.e., virtue) of care in its resolution. Erikson suggested that women, like men, experience a midlife generativity crisis, which results to some extent from age-related social pressures to make a contribution to the next generation. This crisis results in a capacity and commitment to care for ideas, cultural products, institutions, values, and other people (Stewart et al., 2001).

Generativity has only recently been widely discussed. It refers not only to bearing and nurturing children but also includes creativity (i.e., the production of new works and things) and the generation of new ideas. Thus, generativity includes both creating and caring (De St. Aubin et al., 2004). Conventional gender patterns of generativity have changed due to substantial changes in gender roles over time, including the increased vocational aspirations of women and the increased domestic responsibilities of men. Feminists have challenged traditional definitions of generativity as a result of these new conceptions of adult development (De St. Aubin et al., 2004).

Researchers have found a number of differences between middle-aged women and men. The most profound difference in attitude between men and women at middle age is that women are twice as likely as men to be hopeful about the future. More and more women see midlife not as a crisis, but rather as a challenge, or, on a more positive note, as an opportunity to better themselves. They also have a more powerful urge to help others or to make a contribution to some larger good. Women are typically more willing than men at midlife to consider trying something completely new in a search for greater flexibility, challenge, or satisfaction. They are more likely to be optimistic, despite obstacles due to aging. Optimism in middle-aged women takes many forms. Women at midlife believe that they will stay healthy longer than women of previous generations. They are joining gyms at twice the rate of their male peers (Gibbs, 2005). In addition, full-time college enrollment by older women rose to 31% in the past decade (Gibbs, 2005). The National Center on Women & Aging at Brandeis University (as cited in Gibbs, 2005) found that women age 50 and older said that they feel happier about getting older than they had anticipated. Thus, women at midlife feel more confident about their coping skills, which enhances their sense of mastery of life.

Why Midlife and Beyond Is a Time of Empowerment

The responses to our empowerment questionnaire correspond to published research and indicate the same conclusion: Midlife and beyond can be a particularly empowering period in a woman's life. This reality is in opposition to the stereotypes that are present in the culture about this time in women's lives. A recent article in *Time* magazine (Gibbs, 2005) focused on how midlife women in this generation are taking advantage of this critical life period in order to reinvent themselves. Rather than falling prey to the obstacles of midlife, women are figuring out how to turn challenges into opportunities. As a result of higher incomes, better education, and considerable experience at managing multiple roles, women may actually realize that there has never been a better time than now to have a "midlife crisis." Because such a large cluster of women are experiencing middle age (i.e., there are roughly 43 million American women ages 40 to 60), some rules may have to be rewritten and boundaries shifted to accommodate them. The word "crisis" may not apply to midlife for women in this generation because they are creating a new model for what midlife might look like.

Gibbs (2005) found that women, more specifically, middle and upper middle class and professional women, from their 50s on, often experience the most fruitful and satisfying period of life. Many women, at this time of their lives, realize skills and strengths that were never before tapped or exercised. Others experience this period as one of tremendous growth, and they frequently redefine their personalities. In some cases, occupational and social pursuits are picked up where they had been left off for years due to marriage and familial responsibilities. Women have a great deal to look forward to during this exciting period in their lives such as travel, work, sociability, and study. The midlife years are a time to try new things, to go to places never visited before, and to do things not done earlier. Books and magazine articles urge women at about age 50 to take the time to think seriously about what is most important to them and what they want to accomplish with the rest of their lives.

Staying involved in professional organizations and volunteering are ways for older women to have an influence and a voice. Of course, one probably has the most impact with continuing professional involvement. The vast majority of women who are chairs of academic departments, high level executives, and owners of small businesses are also in this age bracket.

This is also a wonderful time of opportunity and freedom, and many women exert their influence politically. Currently, the number of midlife women in the population is larger than ever, which means that there is an increasingly important role for older women in public life. Many older women activists consider feminism broadly in this context and perceive their activities as a means of nurturing others. Women in their 50s and beyond are in perfect positions to make great impacts on local, national, and even worldwide levels. For example, nearly all of the women in the United States Congress are at least 50 years old (Congressional Research Service, 2004).

Times are changing for women in general, and "the daughters of today's women" are more likely than their mothers to be well-educated, to have explored several personal options, and to have had long years of employment experiences. Therefore, they are more likely, when grey hair and wrinkles appear, to resist being pushed aside by younger people (Lott, 1987). Currently, older active women in the United States and worldwide can and do have an impact on the world around them, at least in part by virtue of their age. Women gain personal power, prestige, and influence as they grow older. The perceived balance of interpersonal power in the latter half of women's lives increases in favor of older women. This increase is also apparent in terms of equality between men and women during the later stages of a woman's development. It is interesting that it is the social status of a woman that impacts on her power, and it is those women who have achieved a higher social status who can expect to have a greater amount of perceived power in their middle and later years (Todd et al., 1990). Conditions for gifted women during their 50s and beyond are particularly positive.

Some women say that life "begins" at 50, and it is not uncommon for women at midlife and even later to discover new talents and interests and employ them successfully (Allington & Troll, 1984). One study (Mitchell & Helson, 1990) indicated that women in their early 50s gave higher satisfaction ratings to their lives than did either older or younger women. An increasing number of women are beginning or returning to college or work in middle or older adulthood after years of devoting their lives exclusively to their families. These women are referred to as "reentry" women. Despite the obstacles these women face, reentry women tend to do very well in their pursuits. In college, they work hard and participate actively in their education. Research (De Groot, 1980) shows that women who attend college at an older age are more assertive and, as such, expect and receive more spousal support, which increases the likelihood of their success. Middle-aged women also function effectively in the workplace and experience great job satisfaction. This is particularly true for those in "careers" as opposed to those with "jobs." In one study (Coleman & Antonucci, 1983) older women in the workforce reported experiencing greater psychological well-being, self-esteem, and health than did their homemaker counterparts. These findings attest to the possibilities and opportunities that arise during midlife for women. The population of reentry women is likely to increase as life spans grow longer and good health care continues longer in life.

All of these factors combine to make midlife and beyond a fruitful and productive time in women's lives, one that breeds empowerment. Women perceive themselves as intelligent, assertive, and determined in middle age, and they are serious about the task of empowering themselves and others (Babladelis, 1999). Women in midlife are geared through family, economic, and social factors to be able to focus on their own needs, and they often have the means to ascertain them successfully.

The 50s onward appears to be almost a golden age for certain women. Studies (e.g., Mitchell & Helson, 1990) have shown that women feel secure, enjoy good health, and experience a fairly autonomous and androgynous period of time. College educated women in their early 50s who were polled as to their quality of life and current life satisfaction rated their lives as "first-rate" (Mitchell & Helson, 1990). Good health and increased income during these years also contribute to feelings of security, greater self-confidence, involvement, and breadth of personality by women who are older. Considering the 50s onward as the empowering prime of life for women is an appropriate classification (Mitchell & Helson, 1990).

The "Empty Nest" Syndrome

The effects of the so-called empty nest syndrome (i.e., when children leave home) vary from person to person. Midlife women who work can enjoy benefits such as professional development, financial autonomy, intellectual stimulation, an expanded social group, and a sense of self-independent of the family. These women may associate an empty nest with a sense of relief and an opportunity for greater marital satisfaction (Rollins, 1989). As relationships mature during midlife, tender feelings of affection and loyalty tend to replace passion and sexual intimacy as a main focus (Reedy et al., 1981). Thus, some marriages, although turbulent in early adulthood, turn out to be better adjusted during middle adulthood. Many women view their children's departure as an overall positive event, even if they have mixed emotions about it (Troll, 1989). The empty nest is really only problematic for those women whose lives revolve around their children to the exclusion of outside interests and activities. This may suggest that in today's day and age, with many more than one-half of American women working outside the home and building their own careers, the empty nest syndrome is becoming less and less common.

Conceptions of Empowerment: Race, Class, and Cross-cultural Factors

It is important to include in any discussion about empowerment, the socially bound structures of inequality that make empowerment more or less difficult for certain groups of women. Within the United States, discrimination based on race, class, and culture all work against women of these groups, making empowerment a critical force in their lives but a challenging one to achieve.

Empowerment and Race

In addition to sex discrimination, African American women must mediate and overcome the disadvantages placed on them due to race (Parker, 2003). Therefore, Women of Color must mediate different levels of oppression, which can make empowerment doubly challenging in these women's lives.

In the process of defending against the sexism and racism of society, African American women have developed strategies and processes of their own in order to empower themselves. Unlike European American women who are faced only with patriarchal systems of domination, African American women are part of that reality but also are faced with racist systems of domination. This duality has created the need for African American women to empower themselves in unique ways.

A review of the literature (Parker, 2003) shows that there are five themes specific to midlife African American women and their empowerment. These are: developing and using voice, being self-defined, being self-determined, connecting and building community, and seeking spirituality and regeneration. African American women have developed a Black feminist standpoint, which conceptualizes self-definition and self-determination as the power to name and decide one's own destiny. Community, spirituality, and speaking out against oppression have also been used as tools and methods through which to attain empowerment.

Especially in working contexts, African American women must "negotiate and reconcile the contradictions separating internally defined images of self as African American women whose identities are (re)produced through patriarchal systems of domination and subordination" (Parker, 2003, p. 262). It is this process of negotiating identities that has given African American women unique ways of empowering themselves. They actively strive to use the strategies mentioned above to work against the stereotypes that patriarchal society has developed.

The empowerment model is a model of social change and therapeutic intervention that focuses on promoting assets, strengths, and resilience in people (Querimit & Conner, 2003). This has important implications for Women of Color in midlife and beyond. Quermit and Conner (2003) studied this model in youth of Color but many comparisons can be made to older Women of Color as well. Women over 50 still must overcome social inequality, but now they have achieved more skills and assets on which to rely. They can depend upon these developed strengths in order to empower themselves, despite the social inequalities and oppression in their lives. In this way, age becomes a mediating factor and an aid in empowering older Women of Color.

The following is a case example of an African woman who used many of the strategies noted above to empower herself. Ellen Johnson-Sirleaf, President of Liberia, is a prime example of a woman over 50 who promotes empowerment for women. Elected by a stunning 60% of the vote in November 2005 to become the first female elected leader in Africa's history, Johnson-Sirleaf now has the responsibility of mending her broken country. A Harvard graduate in economics, Johnson-Sirleaf is currently tackling the economic and social problems in her country. Born to two Liberian parents who were adopted by American Liberians living in the United States, she was instilled with a sense of duty and honesty. On the way, however, she has not forgotten issues important to the women of her country. She is working to raise public consciousness about issues of wife abuse, rape, and women's inheritance of property. A rape victim herself, she, along with a group of lawyers, has worked to enact laws that ensure that rapists will be penalized with stricter sentences. According to Hammer (2006), Johnson-Sirleaf is one of the growing number of women in Africa who are climbing to power and working toward women's empowerment initiatives. African women are "breaking the male stranglehold on national legislation, cabinets, courts, and other government institutions. They're making laws, changing attitudes, inspiring other women to follow them" (Hammer, 2006, p. 32). In other words, Johnson-Sirleaf embodies the concept of the empowerment of women.

Empowerment and Class

The discussion of class is clearly related to empowerment. Many Women of Color are also living in poverty or struggling to provide for themselves and their families.

Women immigrants, and women of all ethnicities born into families below the poverty line, report that monetary disadvantage has led to part of the disempowerment that they experience (Darlington & Mulvaney, 2003). Darlington and Mulvaney (2003) distributed a questionnaire to 25 women who identified themselves as Hispanic, Cuban American, Spanish, White Spanish, White Cuban American, and "multi." Questions were aimed at determining these women's view of power and empowerment in the United States. Some women's statements make clear the connection between class and empowerment. As a response to what they thought power meant in the United States today, one women stated that power in American society is "to be White and to have money" (all quotes p. 131). Other responses included that power is "wealth, it seems only rich people are powerful," "I think power is related to wealth; it's also related to how much you've got in terms of what you drive and what you wear," and "Power is viewed as a tool for control." In terms of power definitions in Latin American countries, these women said that power was also related to control. One woman said that power is "To be of high class, have studied in good private schools, and to come from a wealthy family."

Andrews et al. (2003) studied the conceptualization of empowerment by women in poverty and lower socioeconomic classes, specifically from the southern United States. These women had to endure geographic isolation, unemployment, low educational attainment, and limited access to services. Participants' comments about a fictitious woman named Angela and her life story were audiotaped for analysis to capture the women's beliefs about what methods are possible for Angela to use to break free from the difficult situation in which she finds herself (Angela is poor with few resources). The women were asked to comment about Angela's life and about her strengths and limitations. Empowerment was woven into their answers, and most women thought that Angela needed to take control of her life, despite the challenges with which she is confronted due to her class status. Their conceptions of empowerment were in strong relation to notions of class and the need to break free from the trouble that low socioeconomic status creates (i.e., to empower oneself). There were themes in their responses of optimism, persistence, ability to let go, ability to seek and accept help, and spirituality. Their responses indicated that empowering attributes were closely related to interpersonal and environmental factors and were not in isolation to what was experienced day to day.

The results of that study make it clear that class is a large consideration in women's conceptions of who is empowered and who is not. In both the United States and in immigrants' countries of origin, the upper classes have more power, and they are "entitled" to greater advantages that the society has to offer. In the United States and elsewhere, class is, therefore, also related to empowerment, in that lower classes must strive harder to empower themselves in a society that is structurally skewed against them. Becker et al. (2004) also sought to operationalize individual notions of empowerment in a sample of advocates working with low-income mothers. Overall, these authors used the term empowerment outright as "setting goals, gathering information, defining needs, and making and implementing decisions" (p. 332). All of these were ways in which the women could empower themselves and, in doing this, help to alleviate the pressures put on them by their class status.

Empowerment and Cross-cultural Factors

It is important to bear in mind that notions of empowerment vary with culture and ethnic background. Agency and self-sufficiency are often used as theoretical indicators and measures of "successful" aging and quality of life. Along these lines, success is associated with individual potential, or with the ability to adapt to the challenges of getting older. However, this is highly problematic for two reasons. First of all, these notions are derived from dominant Euro-American conceptions of what constitutes power, which are often associated with notions of independence and autonomy that are Western-specific. Such concepts vary according to time and space and confer different meanings across different ethnicities, cultures, and historical time periods. Second, existing knowledge of what constitutes autonomy, independence, agency, and empowerment in later life tends to be uncritically and universally applied, which results in the endorsement of dominant values and perceptions (Wray, 2004). Instead, researchers should investigate how diverse social, cultural, and historical backgrounds shape perceptions and experiences of successful aging. Specifically, the impact of cultural and ethnic affiliation on notions of agency, empowerment, and disempowerment should be assessed. To understand what constitutes agency and empowerment necessitates an analysis of the values, beliefs, and norms that distinguish cultural groupings.

It is also important to note that various countries have different cultural levels of gender empowerment. In 2004, the United Nations Development Program ranked 78 countries based on number of seats in Parliament held by women, the number of female officials and managers, the number of female professional and technical workers, and the ratio of estimated women's to men's earned income. Results indicated that Norway attained the highest gender empowerment rank, the United States was 14th, Japan was 38th, and Saudi Arabia was 77th (United Nations Development Program, 2004). See Table 10.1.

Wray (2004) investigated experiences of agency, empowerment, and disempowerment in 170 British women between 60- and 80-years-old. These women came from a wide range of ethnic backgrounds, which affected their perceptions of what constituted agency and control in their lives. For instance, quality of life may be defined in a number of ways: medical/health factors, social support, personal development and fulfillment, income, and relations with others. However, results indicated that there was some agreement across groups that good health was an important quality of life issue. The majority regarded having a degree of control over their health and agility as central to agency and autonomy. Yet, despite this, health-related problems (e.g., asthma, diabetes, arthritis) did not prevent the women from getting on with and enjoying their lives (Wray, 2004). In addition, religious and spiritual beliefs were an important factor that influenced their quality of life. However, differences emerged between ethnic groups in the significance attached to beliefs as sources of collective agency and empowerment. The majority

TABLE 10.1. Gender empowerment by country.

Country	Gender empowerment measure (GEM) rank	Seats in parliament held by women (% of total)	Female legislators senior officials and managers (% of total)	Female professional and technical workers (% of total)	Ratio of estimated women's to men's earned income
Norway	1	36.4	28	49	0.74
Canada	10	23.6	34	54	0.63
New Zealand	11	28.3	38	52	0.69
Austria	13	30.6	29	48	0.36
United States	14	14.0	46	55	0.62
Mexico	34	21.2	25	40	0.38
Japan	38	9.9	10	46	0.46
Venezuela	61	9.7	27	61	0.41
Republic of Korea	68	5.9	5	34	0.46
Pakistan	64	20.8	9	26	0.33
Saudi Arabia	77	0.0	1	31	0.21

Source: (United Nations Development Program, 2004).

spoke of the happiness, sense of well-being, belongingness, hope, and empowerment that they derived from their beliefs and how these feelings emerged in their daily lives.

Overall, interdependence was an important source of empowerment and agency (Wray, 2004). Having a continuing role to play in the lives of their children contributed feelings of authority, self-worth, and power. Here, power is an aspect of interdependency and reciprocity rather than of independence and self-sufficiency. The absence of this type of collaborative reciprocity and/or the loss of the parenting role was cited as potentially disempowering across ethnic groups. Grandparenting was also perceived differently across culture. For some African Caribbean and Dominican women, and for a small number of White British women, grandparenting provided opportunities to act autonomously. For other women, child-care and domestic responsibilities were viewed in a more negative light. Some British Muslim women spoke of their preference to live apart from their children due to a desire for freedom from familial responsibilities and for independence. There was evidence to suggest that a number of British Pakistani and Indian women lived alone and preferred it that way. Women living in extended families often found their living arrangements to be both empowering and disempowering. On the one hand, playing an active role as a family member was viewed in a positive manner. Alternatively, others viewed living with offspring as undesirable due to their need for privacy or freedom from responsibilities and obligations.

Overall, Wray (2004) demonstrated that women from different backgrounds use different strategies to pursue active lives and to remain in control as they grow older. Thus, what constitutes agency and empowerment for women in mid and later life is a question that generates a variety of responses, all of which deserve equal attention and investigation.

Organizations That Promote Empowerment

As we have seen previously, midlife and older women tend to participate more actively in politics and in organized efforts for social change. Some older women view their efforts as connected to feminism (Garland, 1988). In fact, midlife women have been instrumental in improving their positions through organizations like the Gray Panthers, the National Organization for Women (NOW), the Association for Women in Psychology (AWP), and groups connected to the United Nations.

The National Organization for Women (NOW)

NOW is the largest organization of feminist activists in the United States, with 500,000 contributing members and 550 chapters in all 50 states and the District of Columbia. NOW has decades of experience in political advocacy, training local activists, and providing their members with the resources to organize and to be strong advocates for women's rights. NOW's goal is to take action in order to bring about equality for all women. Activists strive for the "feminization of power" and support women's rights candidates for election to federal, state, and local governments. NOW works to eliminate discrimination and harassment in the workplace, the schools, the justice system, and all other sectors of society; to secure abortion, birth control, and other reproductive rights for all women; to end all forms of violence against women; to eradicate racism, sexism, and homophobia; and to promote equality and justice in our society. NOW's actions have greatly contributed to extensive changes that have put more women in political posts. NOW's efforts have also increased educational, employment, and business opportunities for women. In addition, NOW has worked for stricter laws against violence, harassment, and discrimination against women. NOW's official priorities are to win economic equality and secure it with an amendment to the U.S. constitution that will guarantee equal rights for women; to champion abortion rights, reproductive freedom, and other women's health issues; to oppose racism and fight bigotry against lesbians and gay men; and to end violence against women. Now activists use both traditional and nontraditional means to push for social change. They do extensive electoral and lobbying work, and they bring lawsuits. They organize mass marches, rallies, pickets, nonviolent civil disobedience, and immediate, responsive "zap" actions (National Organization for Women, 2006).

The Gray Panthers

The Gray Panthers is a national intergenerational grassroots organization that was founded by older people. Members strive to achieve progressive social change in a variety of domains that affect people of all ages. Such issues include antidiscrimination, social and economic justice, affordable housing, universal health care, peace, educational improvement, and environmental preservation. Gray Panthers believe that, in an interdependent world, the welfare of all is achieved by policies that preserve peace, heal the wounded environment, and respect the rights of all individuals to share in determining policy. Furthermore, they seek to unite young, old, women, and men of all ethnic, racial, and economic backgrounds for the study and promotion of social justice. They reason that governments exist in order to facilitate the achievement of social justice for all (Gray Panthers, 2006).

Association for Women in Psychology (AWP)

Other organizations are more focused on particular issues. For instance, the AWP was founded in 1969 at the American Psychological Association's (APA) annual convention; however it operates outside of the APA's organizational structure and maintains a broader-than-psychology membership and vision. AWP sponsors regional and national conferences on feminist psychology as well as several annual awards. They frequently collaborate with other organizations to promote a feminist approach to research, teaching, and mental health, and they maintain an active liaison program with other feminist and psychological organizations. AWP has been an official non-governmental organization (NGO) of the United Nations since 1976 and has participated in international conferences.

AWP is a not-for-profit scientific and educational organization committed to encouraging feminist psychological research, theory, and activism. AWP has a strong a history of supporting and celebrating differences, deepening challenges, and experiencing growth as feminists. AWP is devoted to reevaluating and reformulating the role that psychology and the mental health field generally play within women's lives. They seek to act responsively and sensitively with regard to women by challenging the unquestioned assumptions, research traditions, theoretical commitments, clinical and professional practices, and institutional and societal structures that limit the understanding, treatment, professional attainment, and self-determination of women and men, or that contribute to unwelcome divisions between women based on race, ethnicity, age, social class, sexual orientation, or religious affiliation. Thus, AWP's role includes the education and sensitization of mental health professionals, the encouragement and recognition of women's concerns and those who promote them, the reconceptualization and expansion of perspectives within psychology, advocacy and critique regarding professional and institutional practices, and the provision of opportunities for creative feminist contributions and the dissemination of feminist ideas (Association for Women in Psychology, 2006).

Lobbying by AWP was directly responsible for the establishment of the Society for the Psychology of Women (APA Division 35) in 1973. Joint AWP and Division 35 efforts resulted in the establishment of a Women's Program Office at APA's national headquarters. The AWP agenda includes efforts to eliminate racism in public and private organizations. One goal of the association is to make people aware of the interface between gender and race in the psychology of women. One of AWP's primary purposes is feminist activism. AWP is devoted to achieving various objectives: (1) challenging unfounded assumptions about the psychological "natures" of women and men; (2) encouraging feminist psychological research on sex and gender; (3) combating the oppression of Women of Color; (4) developing a feminist model of psychotherapy; (5) achieving equality for women within the profession of psychology and allied disciplines; (6) promoting unity among women of all races, ages, social classes, sexual orientations, physical abilities, and religions; (7) sensitizing the public and the profession to the psychological, social, political, and economic problems of women; (8) helping women to create individual sexual identities; and (9) encouraging research on issues of concern to Women of Color.

American Psychological Association—Division 35—Society for the Psychology of Women

Division 35 was founded in 1973 in order to focus on the psychology of women. Today, there are over 2400 members. The Society is "devoted to providing an organizational base for all feminists, women, and men of all national origins who are interested in teaching, research or practice in the psychology of women" (American Psychological Association, 2005). The purpose of Division 35 is to promote feminist research, theories, education, and practice; to encourage scholarship on the social construction of gender relations across multicultural contexts; to apply feminist scholarship to transforming the knowledge base of psychology; and to advocate action toward public policies that advance equality. Empowerment is, therefore, very highly linked to the goals and purpose of this division within APA. Through many different media, women are encouraged to strive toward empowerment and also to facilitate the way for structural changes to be made to help achieve empowerment for future generations.

The United Nations

An international organization that can facilitate the advancement of empowerment for the world's women is the United Nations. The UN plays a central role in the promotion of peace and security, development, and human rights around the world. Since its founding, the UN has been working to affirm the fundamental equality of all people and to counter discrimination in all its forms. Through UN efforts, governments have concluded many multilateral agreements that make the world a safer, healthier place with greater opportunity and justice *for all of us*. The United Nations provides the means to help resolve international conflicts and formulate policies on matters that affect everyone. At the UN, all the member states—large and small, rich and poor, with different political views and social systems—have a voice and a vote in this process (United Nations, 2006). One of the UN's central mandates is the promotion of higher standards of living, full employment, and conditions of economic and social progress and development. As much as 70% of the work of the UN system is devoted to accomplishing this mandate. Guiding the work is the belief that eradicating poverty and improving the well-being of people everywhere are necessary steps in creating conditions for lasting world peace. The UN and its agencies, including the World Bank and the UN Development Programme, are the premier vehicles for furthering development in poorer countries.

The millennium development goals (MDGs,), issued by the UN Secretary General Kofi Annan in 2001, are a "roadmap" for implementing the Millennium Declaration, which was presented at the September 2000 UN Millennium Summit. The Millennium Declaration reflects widespread international recognition that the empowerment of women and the achievement of gender equality are issues of human rights and social justice. Equality and women's empowerment are fundamental to the achievement of all of the MDGs, whether it is the eradication of poverty, protection of the environment, or access to healthcare. Attempts to meet the MDGs without integrating gender equality would both raise the cost and diminish the success. Because the MDGs are mutually reinforcing, success in attaining the goals will have positive effects on gender equality, just as advancement toward gender equality in any one domain will help to promote each of the other goals (Women's Environment & Development Organization, 2004).

By the year 2015, all 191 UN Member States have pledged to meet the MDG goals. The eight MDGs include: (1) eradicate extreme poverty and hunger; (2) achieve universal primary education; (3) promote gender equality and empower women; (4) reduce child mortality; (5) improve maternal healthcare; (6) combat HIV/AIDS, malaria, and other diseases; (7) ensure environmental sustainability; and (8) develop a global partnership development (Millennium Project, 2006).

Goal #3 makes clear the importance of activating a comprehensive, rather than a piecemeal, program to advance gender equality. Accordingly, Goal #3 encompasses gender equality in all aspects of women's lives—gender-based violence, cultural stereotypes, trafficking and prostitution, armed conflict, political life, laws and legal status, government structures, the media, education, employment, health care, family planning, poverty, the environment, rural life, and marriage and family relations. The full range of measures that must be taken to achieve gender equality and women's empowerment have already been comprehensively mapped out in the Convention on the Elimination of All Forms of Discrimination against Women (CEDAW) and the Beijing Platform for Action, as well as in major provisions of other international instruments and conference documents (UNIFEM, 2004).

In addition to the UN's international policy programs and organizations, the NGOs within the UN promote social awareness and activism of various issues. Two specific NGOs, the committee on the status of women and the committee on ageing, are active in promoting the empowerment of women. The committee on the status of women, specifically the sub-committee of older women (SCOW), is a group of women, primarily over 50, who promote issues and education of issues that are relevant to women in this age group. The NGO committee on the status of women (NGO CSW) was founded after the UN general assembly proclaimed 1975 as the International Women's Year and recommended that international action be intensified to: promote equality between men and women; ensure full integration of women in the total development effort; and recognize the importance of women's increasing contribution to the development of friendly relations and cooperation among states; and to strengthen world peace. The NGO CSW New York provides a forum for exchange of information, education, and awareness and for substantive discussion on issues and policies related to women under consideration by the United Nations as well as other relevant women-related studies and programs (Women's United Nations Report Program & Network, n.d.). SCOW prepares statements and prepares events related to issues and changes that need to be made on behalf of older women. The women in these committees exemplify empowerment at its best: Women work together to promote key issues and, in doing, so they affect positive change for women of all ages. The NGO Committee on Ageing's work also coincides with the empowerment of women. This NGO works to promote issues relevant to older persons, many of whom are women.

UNIFEM, or the United Nations' Development Fund for Women, works on behalf of women from all countries of the world. It provides financial and technical assistance to innovative programs and strategies to foster women's empowerment and gender equality. Specifically, the UNIFEM Arab States Regional Office's projects and programs target many different aspects of women's lives in this region, such as economic rights, human rights, and involvement in the political process. UNIFEM programs promote women's leadership in all sectors, with the goal of giving women an equal voice in shaping the policies that affect their lives and choices. Through its projects and activities, UNIFEM aims to achieve the following objectives to support women's leadership: (1) peace and security—strengthening gender focus in prevention, making gender perspectives central to peace processes, and supporting gender justice in postconflict peace-building; (2) gender justice—women's empowerment and equal participation in leadership and political decision making are necessary elements for ensuring that gender equality is integrated into policy making and constitutional, electoral, and judicial reform (UNIFEM, 2004).

Women and Leadership: Using Leadership to Empower Others

Women have increasingly gained greater leadership roles in organizations and thus have had a greater impact on corporate strategy. The management literature suggests that the values of future organizations may suit women to a greater degree than was the case for women in the past (Colwill & Townsend, 1999). Self-knowledge, building relationships, facilitation skills, and empowering others are emerging as essential skills for all managers. These skills are increasingly identified as the central elements for successful executives, a movement away from the traditional male autocrat of the 1970s. Research (Colwill & Townsend, 1999) has shown that many characteristics identified as "good management skills" are also characteristics ascribed to "traditional women." Many of these good managerial abilities relate to communication patterns. For instance, overall, women value communication and relationships, such as working together toward a common purpose, and understanding others (Colwill & Townsend, 1999). Women are more exploratory and less instrumental in their communication than men are. They are more likely to communicate issues that are judged unnecessary by men, but, in doing so, they can impart a broader understanding to others (Colwill & Townsend, 1999).

Merely being recognized as a leader does not make one either powerful or empowering. For example, Queen Elizabeth II of the United Kingdom and Northern Ireland, Queen Margrethe II of Denmark, and Queen Beatrix Wilhelmina Armgard of the Netherlands are primarily figureheads. Other leaders are powerful or have been powerful but not empowering, such as Margaret Thatcher, Indira Gandhi, and Condoleezza Rice. Women leaders who have worked to empower other women include Susan B. Anthony, Betty Freidan, Gloria Steinem, Hillary Rodham Clinton, Oprah Winfrey, and Donna Shalala, President of the University of Miami and former Secretary of the U.S. Department of Health and Human Services. Although Hillary Clinton became known as the First Lady of the United States, it was not until she was into her 50s that she was elected a U.S. senator in her own right.

Empowerment is demonstrated not only in the political sphere but in others as well. Take the American painter, Grandma Moses, as she is commonly called. Anna May Robertson Moses was the third of 10 children, and she was encouraged as a child by her father to paint and draw. She worked on a neighboring farm from the age of 12 until her marriage to Thomas Salmon Moses in 1887. While living on the farm that the couple owned and worked together, Grandma Moses decorated certain objects in her home with painted scenes, but it was only in her 70s, with no prior artistic training or formal classes that she started to paint in oils. Her paintings are on display in museums worldwide and have brought her to the forefront as an example of what can be accomplished by women over 50 (ArtCyclopedia, 2005).

According to Pillai (1995), empowerment is an active multidimensional process that enables women to realize their full identity and power in all spheres of life. Empowerment for women involves having a say and being listened to as well as being able to create from a woman's perspective. Empowerment insists that women be appreciated and acknowledged for who they are and what they do. Once recognized, they are more effective in their future endeavors. They develop a capacity to face the social facts of their actual situation boldly. They are able to come to a better understanding of themselves and their circumstances once they examine the truth of their lives. An empowered woman becomes free of social, cultural, and, perhaps most important, psychological barriers (Pillai, 1995).

Just as many individuals are not entirely self-actualized according to Maslow's theory, many individuals also are not fully empowered (Maslow, 1943). There are various steps that women can take in order to become more empowered. Women can

- gain control of our lives (e.g., through sufficient education, self-exploration, finding interests, skill development, choosing a satisfying career and lifestyle, receiving therapy);
- gain awareness about our own situations, our rights, and available opportunities;
- bring our capabilities to optimum use;

- lead fulfilling lives;
- enhance confidence, self-esteem, self-respect, and self-dignity;
- gain economic independence and control our own resources;
- capacity building and skill development, especially the ability to plan, make decisions, organize, and carry out activities;
- learn to deal with the people and situations/institutions around us;
- participate in decision making at home, in the local community, and in the greater society;
- learn from our past and build our future;
- develop an assertive belief system;
- build relationships (e.g., romantic, friendship, career networks);
- move from passive inaction to active participation;
- be able to influence choices and decisions that affect the whole society;
- be organized and gain respect as equal citizens and human beings with contributions to make;
- move beyond ourselves and contribute toward the empowerment of others;
- cooperate with other women toward a common good.

Conclusions

Empowerment is an issue that is relevant to women of all socioeconomic classes, races, and cultures. It is particularly pertinent in any discussion of women at midlife, considering that middle class women of this age group frequently have the necessary capabilities needed to make positive changes in their lives and to turn the balance of power in their favor. There are various steps to empowerment that these women have used. Many have been successful at gaining control of their lives, enhancing their confidence and self-esteem, gaining awareness of their situation, and developing an assertive belief system. However, some women, particularly those of lower socioeconomic status or ethnic minorities who are discriminated against, find themselves in a particularly challenging situation when it comes to empowerment. Societal structures and discrimination make it exponentially difficult, but not necessarily impossible, to follow these steps to empowerment for these women.

One critical component to empowerment is moving beyond ourselves toward the empowerment of others. Empowerment must be viewed not only as personal empowerment, but also as the empowerment of other women. Women must work toward the empowerment of all women, and one way to support this is to cooperate with other women toward a common good. One way that this has been accomplished is through the establishment of groups and organizations that have been constructed to help women empower themselves, such as NOW, AWP, and the Gray Panthers.

In addition, in the political sphere, world policy is finally beginning to support the empowerment of women by encouraging policies that empower women and give them the much needed resources to help fight poverty, discrimination, and inequality. Women in midlife can be examples of the productive, able, and resourceful qualities that most women possess. With increased support from organizations and government, as well as with the increased cooperative participation of women of all ages, women's empowerment will continue to increase.

Overall, women over 50 are in a prime period in their lives where they can exemplify and expand empowerment for themselves and other women. Now that the children have grown up and left the house, women have more time to dedicate to efforts to enhance their lives and their societies. They also have more financial resources at their disposal and the means to set goals and attain them. This includes an increased sense of confidence, which comes with age and experience. More life experience gives women key assets to learn new strategies and the personal ability to put these strategies into effect. Women over 50 have many key elements in place to continue to promote the empowerment of themselves as well as that of other women of all ages.

Acknowledgment. We thank Lani Sherman for her assistance with the questionnaire distribution.

References

Allington, D.E., and Troll, L.E. (1984). Social change and equality: The roles of women and economics. In G. Baruch and J. Brooks-Gunn (Eds.), *Women in Midlife* (pp. 181–202). New York: Plenum.

American Heritage Dictionary of the English Language (4th ed.). (2000) Boston: Houghton Mifflin.

American Psychological Association. (2005). *Division 35—Society for the Psychology of Women.* Retrieved October 4, 2005, from http://www.apa.org/about/ division/div35 .html.

Andrews, A.B., Guadalupe, J.L., and Bolden, E. (2003). Faith, hope and mutual support: Paths to empowerment as perceived by women in poverty. *Journal of Social Work Research and Evaluation, 4*, 5–18.

ArtCycylopedia (2005). *Grandma Moses.* Retrieved from http://www.artcyclopedia.com/artists/moses_grandma.html.

Association for Women in Psychology. (2006). *The Association for Women in Psychology.* Retrieved from www.awpsych.org.

Babladelis, G. (1999). Autonomy in the middle years. In M.B. Nadien and F.L. Denmark (Eds.), *Females and Autonomy—A Lifespan Perspective* (pp. 101–129). Boston: Allyn & Bacon.

Becker, J., Kovach, A.C., and Gronseth, D.L. (2004). Individual empowerment: How community health workers operationalize self-determination, self-sufficiency, and decision-making abilities of low income mothers. *Journal of Community Psychology, 32*, 327–342.

Browne, C.V. (1995). Empowerment in social work practice with older women. *Social Work, 40*, 358–364.

Chadiha, L.A., Adams, P., Biegel, D.E., Auslander, W., and Gutierrez, L. (2004). Empowering African American women informal caregivers: A literature synthesis and practice strategies. *Social Work, 49*(1), 97–109.

Chamberlin, J. (1997). A working definition of empowerment. *Psychiatric Rehabilitation Journal, 20*, 43–46.

Coleman, L.M., and Antonucci, T.C. (1983). Impact of work on women at midlife. *Developmental Psychology, 19*, 290–294.
Colwill, J. and Townsend, J. (1999). Women, leadership and information technology. *Journal of Management Development, 18*, 207–213.
Congressional Research Service. (2004). *Membership of the 109th Congress: A Profile*. Retrieved April 5, 2006 from www.er.doe.gov/bes/109th_Congress_1st_Session_CRS_20DEC04.pdf.
De St. Aubin, E., McAdams, D.P., and Kim, T. (2004). *The Generative Society: Caring for Future Generations*. Washington, DC: American Psychological Association.
Darlington, P.S., and Mulvaney, B.M. (2003). *Women, Power, and Ethnicity: Working Toward Reciprocal Empowerment*. New York: Haworth Press.
Denmark, F.L., Rabinowitz, V.C., and Sechzer, J.A. (2005). *Engendering Psychology: Women and Gender Revisited* (2nd ed.). Boston: Allyn and Bacon.
De Groot, S.C. (1980). Female and male returnees: Glimpses of two distinct populations. *Psychology of Women Quarterly, 5*, 358–361.
Garland, A.W. (1988). *Women Activists: Challenging the Abuse of Power*. New York: Feminist Press.
Gibbs, N. (2005, May 16). Midlife crisis? Bring it on! *Time*, pp. 52–66, 63.
Gray Panthers. (2006). *Age and Youth in Action*. Retrieved from www.graypanthers.org.
Hammer, J. (2006, April 3). Healing powers. *Newsweek*, pp. 30–35, 38–39.
Hyde, J.S. (2004). *Half the Human Experience: The Psychology of Women* (4th ed.). Boston: Houghton Mifflin.
Lips, H.M. (2005). *Sex and Gender: An Introduction*. Boston: McGraw Hill.
Lott, B. (1987). *Women's Lives: Themes and Variations in Gender Learning*. Monterey, CA: Brooks/Cole.
Maslow, A.H. (1943). A theory of human motivation. *Psychological Review, 50*, 370–396.
Millennium Project. (2006). *2006: The Year of Action*. Retrieved from http://www.unmillenniumproject.org.
Mitchell, V., and Helson, R. (1990). Women's prime of life: Is it the 50s? *Psychology of Women Quarterly, 14*, 451–470.
National Organization for Women (2006). *About NOW*. Retrieved from http://www.now.org/organization/info.html.
Page, N. and Czuba, C.E. (1999). Empowerment: What is it? *Journal of Extension, 37*(5). Retrieved October 3, 2005 from www.joe.org/joe/1999october/comm1.html.
Parker, P.S. (2003). Resistance and empowerment in raced, gendered, and classed work contexts: The case of African American women. *Communication Yearbook, 27*, 257–291.
Pillai, J.K. (1995). *Women and Empowerment*. New Delhi: Gyan.
Querimit, D.S., and Conner, L.C. (2003). Empowerment psychotherapy with adolescent females of Color. *Journal of Clinical Psychology, 59*, 1215–1224.
Reedy, M.N., Birren, J.E., and Schaie, K.W. (1981). Age and sex differences in satisfying relationships across the life span. *Human Development, 24*, 52–66.
Rollins, B.C. (1989). Marital quality at midlife. In S. Hunter and M. Sundel (Eds.), *Midlife Myths: Issues, Findings, and Practice Implications* (pp. 184–194). Newbury Park, CA: Sage.
Stewart, A.J., Ostrove, J.M., and Helson, R. (2001). Middle aging in women: Patterns of personality change from the 30s to the 50s. *Journal of Adult Development, 8*(1), 23–37.
Todd, J., Friedman, A., and Kariuki, P.W. (1990). Women growing stronger with age: The effect of status in the United States and Kenya. *Psychology of Women Quarterly, 14*, 567–577.

Troll, L.E. (1989). Myths of midlife intergenerational relationships. In S. Hunter and M. Sundel (Eds.), *Midlife Myths: Issues, Findings, and Practice Implications* (pp. 210–231). Newbury Park, CA: Sage.

United Nations. (2006). *About the United Nations: An Introduction to the Structure and Work of the UN*. Retrieved from www.un.org.

United Nations Development Fund for Women. (UNIFEM). (2004). *Pathway to equality: CEDAW, Beijing and the MDGs*. New York: UNIFEM.

United Nations Development Program. (2004). *Human Development Report 2004*. New York: Author.

Women's Environment & Development Organization (WEDO). (2004) *Women's Empowerment: Gender Equality and the Millennium Development Goals: A WEDO Information Action Guide*. New York: Author.

Women's United Nations Report Program & Network (WUNRN). (n.d.).*Organizations: Women's NGOs*. Retrieved from http://www.wunrn.com/organizations/women_ngo/un-ngo_ny.htm.

Wray, S. (2004). What constitutes agency and empowerment for women in later life? *Sociological Review, 52*, 22–38.

Yoder, J.D. (2003). *Women and Gender: Transforming Psychology* (2nd ed.). Upper Saddle River, NJ: Prentice Hall.

Yoder, J.D., and Kahn, A.S. (1992). Toward a feminist understanding of women and power. *Psychology of Women Quarterly, 16*, 381–388.

Index

Advance directives, 70–71
African American women, 189–190
Age
  age group boundaries, 104
  categorization of, 104
  libido and, 105
  power structures, 96, 98
  socio-cultural construct, 97
  well-being and, 104
  "young-old" and, 96
Age concealment, 13
Age identity, 103, 131
Alzheimer's Disease, 61–62
American Association for Retired People (AARP), 79–80, 82–83, 85, 87, 89–91, 177
Americans with Disabilities Act of 1990, 73
Androcentric bias, 32
Anticipatory grief, 152
Arousal, 26–27, 30, 33, 35, 37, 39–41
Arthritis, 14–15, 59–61, 65
Association for Women in Psychology (AWP), 194–195
At risk populations, 86
  disabled, 87
  elderly, 102
  socioeconomic status, 87
  women of color, 57, 81, 118, 172, 189–190
    black, 189
    Hispanic, 86–87, 172, 191
Authenticity/authentic, 19–20, 26, 46, 95, 114

Balance, 21, 84–85, 96, 98, 107, 117, 120
Beauty/beauty ideal, 9, 12–13, 16, 18–19
Bereavement, 157
Black feminist standpoint, 189
Body
  consciousness, 14, 80
  dissatisfaction, 13, 15, 43
  image, 6–9, 12, 14–19, 21, 43, 87, 95, 98
  shape, 19
  size, 10, 12, 13
  surveillance, 11
Body weight
  thinness, 10, 19–20
  weight concerns, 9
  weight consciousness, 8–9
Bone density screening, 59
Bone disease, 59
Brain health, 61–62
Breast cancer, 15, 20, 55, 57
Burden, 119, 140, 151, 154–157

Cardiovascular, 11, 55, 57, 59, 85, 89
Care giving
  aging, 151
  cancer, 152
  dementia, 151, 155–156, 157
  family role, 150–158
  grief, 151–152, 158
  loss, 150–151, 157
  parents, 150
  relationships, 156
  responsibility, 149–151, 153–154
  reversal, 151
  support services, 151, 158
  support, 149–153
  transition, 151
Caregiver strain, 155
Chronic illness
  arthritis, 14–15, 59–61, 65
  cancer, 15, 20
  osteoporosis, 60–61, 84
Committee on Ageing, 197–198
Communal relations, 114
Conflict, 123

Convenience, 8
Convention on the Eliminations of all Forms of Discrimination against women (CEDAW), 197
Coping strategies, 58, 64–66, 72
Cosmetic surgery/plastic surgery, 7
Cross-sex friendships, 113
Culture and empowerment, 192

Depression, 39, 44, 58, 63–65, 72
Discrimination against women, 178
Divorce, 105, 116, 125–126, 133
Dual-career families, 134
Dyspareunia, 28, 30

Eating disorders, 9–10
Empowerment
 class, 189
 cross cultural factors, 190
 definition of, 189
 different countries, 189
Empty nest syndrome, 189
Encouragement, 45, 184, 195
Environmental conditions, 12, 33, 62, 70
Erikson, E.H., 121, 185–186
Estrogens, 54–55, 57–58
Ethnicity hypothesis, 86
Exchange theory/exchange relationships, 114
Exercise & physical activity
 aerobic, 61, 80, 82, 84, 87–90
 anaerobic, 89
 barriers to exercise, 87
 beginning a program, 88
 benefits, 89, 92
 classes, 87, 89–90
 companionship, 114
 duration and frequency, 80
 hectics, 83
 infirm, 83
 maintainers, 83
 mind & body, 83, 85
 overcoming barriers, 87
 socializers, 83
 unmotivated, 83
 weight bearing, 84–85

False friends, 123–124
Family roles, 103, 118, 132–133, 137, 140, 150
Family status, 152
Feminine/femininity, 6, 16, 18, 20
Feminist movement/women's liberation movement, 101–103, 106, 127
Feminist psychologists view, about empowerment, 183–184, 183–184
Feminist therapy, 183
Feminist(s), 10, 20
Flexibility, 19, 42, 83–85, 101
Friendship networks, 116

Gender roles
 diversity of, 115
 expectations, 115
 and life course, 115
 menopause, 115
 reproductive role, 116
 role change, 115
Gender roles, 115
Gender stereotype, 57, 80, 184
Gendered-age
 identity, 101
 lifestyle options, 96, 103
 revised gendered-age roles, 96
 role, 96
 social category, 96
 socio-cultural meanings of, 96
 traditionalism, 97
 and well-being, 97
Generativity, 121, 176
Grandfather, 143
Grandma Moses, 199
Grand mothering style, 135
Grand parenthood, 131–132, 134, 136–139
 functions of, 134
Grand parenting, 131–132, 135, 137–138
Gray Panthers, 194–195

Health care
 poor health care, 81–82
 quality of, 81–82
Heart disease, 54–56
Hormone Replacement Therapy (HRT), 16, 54–55
Hormone replacement, 16, 54–55
Hot flashes, 14, 16, 28
Husbands, 10, 39–41, 113, 116
Hypertension, 68, 81–82
Hypoactive sexual desire, 36

Identity development, 121, 186
Illnesses & disease
 chronic illness, 9, 14, 19, 63–66, 73
 risk factors, 82
Informed consent, 69–70
Interdependence, 96, 117, 183, 193
International Women's Year, 197

Intimacy, 116
Invisibility/invisible women, 7, 19, 21

Johnson–Sirleaf, Ellen, 190
joint replacement, 61

Lesbian(s), 19–20, 42
Life transitions, 125
Locus of control, 11
Loss of desire, 28, 31–32

Marginality hypothesis, 86
Marketing of fitness, 80
Masculine role
    assertiveness, 100
    competence and, 98
    cultural representations of, 99, 107
    instrumentality, 100
    "new" identities, 96, 103–104
    prime of life, 188
Maslow Theory, 199
Media images
    in films/movies, 8
    in magazines, 7–8
Medicalization, 36–37
Menopause, 8–9, 15–19
Mental health, 15, 31, 35, 44
Mental illness, 19, 28
Metabolism, 81, 84, 90
Middle age
    changes in modern society, 132
    and caregiving, 138, 140
    and ethnicity, 166
    friendship after 50
        experience, 119
        roles, 114–116
    and health, 132, 137
    life style, 132
    perceptions of, 136, 139
    socialization to, 138
    stereotype, 135
    as symbol, 131
    transition to, 131, 136–137
    typology, 135
Middle-age, 26, 29–31, 38–39, 79–83, 85, 87–91, 99, 102–103, 105–107, 113, 121, 141–142, 175, 179, 186
Midlife women, 7–12, 14, 17, 19–20
Millennium Development Goals, 197
Mortality, 82–83, 151
Moses, Anna May Robertson, 199
Muscle strength, 83–84, 89

Musculoskeletal, 61, 65, 83, 85, 89
Mutuality, 154, 184

Nutrition
    American diet, 82
New View Campaign, The, 37, 45

Obesity, 81–82, 86
Objectified body consciousness, 14
Off time transition, 137
Older women
    baby boomers, 80, 95, 126, 166, 170
    career advancement, 168
    careers, 53, 88, 134, 140, 167, 170, 172, 174–175, 178
    caregiving, 174
    cohorts, 21, 31, 103, 173, 176
    employment, 164–166
    labor force, 165
    longevity, 140, 170, 174, 178
    occupations, 168
    parentcare, 175
    pensions, 172
    poverty, 178
    retirement, 172, 177–178
    salaries, 166
    sandwich generation, 147, 152, 170
    social security, 174–175
    work force, 165
    work, 164–177
Osteoarthritis & joints, 60–61, 83–84
Osteoporosis & bone strength, 59

Pain management, 148, 152
Patient-provider relationship, 67–68
Perimenopausal, 9
Perimenopause, 9
Physical abilities
    physical fitness, 61, 82–83, 89
Physical activity
    cycling, 80, 89
    gardening, 83, 85, 91
    pilates, 80, 85
    Tai Chi, 85
    walking, 80
    yoga, 80, 85
Physical fitness, 61, 82–84, 89
Physical inactivity
    causes, 86–87
    consequences, 86–87
Politics–political system, 184
Popular media
    double standard, 97, 99

gendered-age identity, 106
  representations, 99, 104, 106–108
  and socio-cultural constructs, 97
Postmenopausal zest, 17
Power
  self support, 103
  and well-being, 103
Power-definition of, 182
Power-over, 183
Power-to, 183
Preference theory, 142
Professional organizations, 187
Proximity, 148

Quality of life, 35, 39, 66, 81

Red Hat society, 126
Re-entry women, 188
Relationship satisfaction, 26, 39–41
Resistance training, 84, 89
Role overload, 154

Safety issues, 41, 87, 173, 175
Same-sex friendships, 112
Sedentary, 82, 85, 89
Self-concept, 8, 11, 97, 118
Self-confidence, 19, 96, 182, 188
Self-efficacy, 11, 65, 100, 155
Self-esteem, 11–12, 15
Self-worth, 11, 193
Sexual desire, 26–27, 29–31
Sexual dysfunction, 34, 36
Sexual response cycle, 27, 33, 45
Sexual responsivity, 29
Sexual revolution
  gendered-age norms, 102
  life-style options, 102
  and well-being, 102
Sexual satisfaction, 30, 35, 39, 41–43, 46
Sexual self esteem, 35
Sexualized society
  cultural standards of, 97
  male domination, 97
Social care, 185
Social class, 37, 92, 115–116, 119
Social construction, 95, 103, 106, 196
Social norms/cultural norms
  appearance comparisons, 19, 107
Social support, 58, 63–64, 66–67, 72

Society for the Psychology of Women (APA Division 35), 195–196
Socioeconomic status, 31, 68, 86
Spirituality, 152, 189–191
Sport
  masters level, 90
Steps to empowerment, 200
Stereotypes
  grandparents of, 135, 184–185
  aging of, 185
Stress, 44, 46, 62–63
  and anxiety, 99
Sub-Committee of Older Women, 197
Support network, 152
Surrogate grandparents, 135

Target Heart Rate (THR), 90
Title IX, 79–80

UN Development Programme, 198
UNIFEM, 198

Vaginal dryness, 16, 27–29, 42
Viagra, 33, 36, 41–42
Vulnerability
  body image, 64, 71
  romance, 64
  sex appeal, 64

Well-being
  and socio-cultural changes, 95–96, 106
  androgyny, 100
  autonomy, 98, 100, 114, 189, 192
  confidence, 99
  fragmented structure of, 95
  gendered balance, 100
  gendered meaning, 96
  in middle life, 98
Widowhood, 116, 125
Women
  education and, 198
  leadership and, 198
Women of color, 57, 81, 86, 118
  Asian/Asian American/Asian-African women, 118
  Black women/African American women, 189–190
  Hispanic women/Latinas, 15, 20, 87, 119, 172
Women's Health Initiative (WHI), 16, 54–55

Printed in the United States
84766LV00002B/201/A